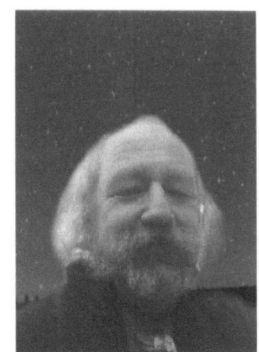

Imprint Lulu.com

Neil Dougan

Perth 6556

West Australia

Neil@neildougan.com

Introduction

The world is in Chaos! Approaches to health, wealth, food, racial and gender inequity are dysfunctional to say the least. It's like living in a house with a fractured foundation. Worn out pillars need to be replaced so the structure does not collapse. The Covid experience served to shine a light on all that is wrong. And now we need thought leaders to emerge in all arenas in order to fix our world.

Even though, if I could I would encourage a change all of society into a more humane Utopian environment. But I cannot. I can however address one societal necessity. And that is medicine.

Modern Medicine, as it has evolved, is overly simplistic, rigid and therefore out of sync with our needs.

Please note, I am not dismissing its many advantages. Instead, I am elaborating on why new paradigms for healing should be added to any medical practitioner's toolbox.

Throughout this book, you will notice several themes repeated in different contexts.

- ✓ Balance
- ✓ Collaboration
- ✓ Cooperation
- ✓ Equality
- ✓ Diversity
- ✓ Harmony
- ✓ Unity

From my perspective, these themes are the pillars of the new world and a new healing modality that fits precisely, like a key designed especially for a lock.

In my work with the candida, of all unlikely sources, I have created a medical model which has been successful in healing hundreds of patients. And these successes come with many differing dysfunctions or diseases. These successes were accomplished assisted by a medical device I created called The Five Brain Coherence Device. The phrase "Five Brains," its meanings and purposes, will become clear as you read this book.

Extensive case studies are included to demonstrate the results.

> The Coherence Device is a tool for assisting a person's neurology around their body into a state something like alpha, the brain activity state that is used by hypnotherapists and meditators alike. There are five major areas within the body with large concentrations of neural ganglia, known as the Five Brains. These are the head brain, the thorax (known also as the heart brain), the abdomen or gut, the pelvis, and the spine. I talk of these as the five brains. The Coherence Device was developed as a key tool in working with the five brains.

It's important to mention a few details about the Candida. They exist throughout the body and operate within a very unique collective called the Hive-Mind. It functions according to a precise set of operating principles

> **The Hive-Mind represents billions if not trillions of cells**
>
> - Directly utilizes all of our mind's information
> - Draws conclusions and does its best to find context.
> - Exists without ranking. These cells equally provide their processing capabilities for the higher good of the collective.
> - Acts in solidarity on behalf of the host.
> - Is eager to collaborate to achieve the best possible outcome for all beings within the human.

Finally, and not of least importance at all, is that the therapy I am about to present is a consciousness-based therapy. As in all healing modalities, consciousness – that of the healer and that of client --plays a huge role in the process. Therefore, I will go into great detail on this most vital element of healing.

PART ONE: Modern Medicine and Its Treatment of Disease

Underlying Premise

In this book, I will be presenting a detailed understanding of this consciousness-based therapy. You will see in the Case Studies a sample of this profound healing potential. But I do not delude myself. My protocol is not the only way to achieve health for you nor your clients. Rather, my core operating principle is *that no one theory is all right or all wrong*.

In every culture, throughout the eons, a theory of medicine and healing has been developed offering its own theory on the derivation of disease and the best approach to overcome it. Chinese, Indian Ayurvedic, European, Western, Indigenous medicinal approaches are the most prominent examples.

The view that the approach of "My theory is right and yours is wrong "is fallacious and narrows the lens through which healing is viewed. Further it doesn't account for the complexity of the human body and all of its systems. From my vantage point, being completely right therefore negating all other views is tyrannical and rigid. It compromises learning and healing. My point of view is to take the best of each and to proceed with whatever works.

Chapter One: Germ Theory and Its Consequences

Modern Medicine and the concept of a disease organism took hold when Louis Pasteur developed Germ Theory in the mid-19th century. This theory identifies microorganisms as the cause of infectious diseases. Disease organisms include bacteria, fungi, (including Candida) and parasites. And which can even be expanded to include viruses, although a virus differs from an organism in ways that are beyond the scope of this book.

Germ theory led to the invaluable life-saving development of sanitation, antiseptics and eventually to antibiotics. Standing out as a core element of Germ Theory that contradicts medicine, as we know it today, is the view that microorganisms are hostile. **This conclusion only makes sense if they are perceived – erroneously or not --as the cause of disease!**

Now modern research has proven there is no such thing as a hostile organism. Microorganisms are part of our innate ecology. They are here to assist the human. Yet the mission of modern medicine as practised in many contries is still to destroy these wrong-fully accused organisms with anti-fungal, anti-parasitic. antibiotic and other anti-microbials.

But the micro-organisms are too smart for that. You see, they replicate rapidly and develop survival mechanisms to protect against the antibiotics. They're the quintessential self-educators and adapters to their environment.

Modern Medicine, Born with Concern

This uneasiness was actually the prophetic leanings of Sir Alexander Fleming who invented the first antibiotic, penicillin.

Without question penicillin saved countless lives. Yet, Fleming expressed tremendous caution about his life-saving invention.

While giving his acceptance speech for the Nobel Prize, on that podium he warned the medical world of the dire potential of antibiotic resistant bacteria. Fleming knew from the start that antibiotics would be over-prescribed and used indiscriminately. And he knew the microorganisms would defend themselves against this class of pharmaceuticals due to the micro-organism's capacity to rapidly replicate.

Fleming was right and the result is that we now have mrsa and other super-bugs that given the right circumstances can readily kill. This is the plague of Modern Medicine today. Yet, Medicine continues to face in the wrong direction by not comprehending that destruction is a failing strategy.

Nevertheless, antibiotics have been invaluable. During WWII, this category of pharmaceuticals prevented amputations, expedited serious wound healing, and saved lives. And it continues to serve a vital purpose in Modern Medicine. Indeed, there are times when antibiotics are absolutely necessary!

Weakening the Immune System

Another deleterious use of many antibiotics, antifungals and other antimicrobials is to utilize approaches that control the immune system. These, in fact, weaken immunity! And they compromise the protocols of a natural medicine practitioner whose goal is to support the body in its natural processes.

As for modern drugs, their performance also runs counter to their intent. They make it harder and harder for the body to self-manage. And they make it harder for natural medicine to succeed.

(Message from the Candida Hive-mind - "We see how the immune system works and we see how you try to copy it with your natural and allopathic medicines, also with your approaches to diet, let alone your use of antibiotics and antifungals and even how you work with subtle medicines and consciousness" – we know these patterns.")

Chapter 2: The Single Cause Approach and Other Misjudgements

A Simplistic View

Another major fault in Modern Medicine is its dedication to searching out the one singular causal factor in disease. The medical research is littered with this reductionist way of viewing the world. Indeed, it is difficult to get your ideas published in a medical journal if you don't follow this approach of reductionist thinking.

We each know people who will talk about how "I went to the doctor and s/he ran all of these blood tests" or something similar. The western medicine perspective has almost no acknowledgement of the complexity of any disease presentation and the involvement of many more factors than a single disease organism.

Most commonly, there will be multiple organisms out of balance, added to multiple systems in the body being out of balance. Yet, the normal allopathic response is to try to simplify a disease presentation down to a single causal factor and if that causal factor is a microbe, then to treat that one organism in a monolithic fashion. If this approach fails, then pharmaceuticals are used to try to control whole classes of microbes. Rarely will modern medicine acknowledge that there are multiple disease vectors in play at once.

This out-dated approach sees the body as disparate parts rather than one whole organism. It takes the stance that the gut is not connected to the brain, that the heart is not connected to the kidneys and so on and so on.

Blind-sighted from what appears to be simple common sense, the modern medicine practitioner is on the pursuit for that one causal factor of a disease manifestation. And feels satisfied when s/he feels they have identified it. The patient is in the position of seeing one doctor for the gastro-intestinal tract, another for their heart, another for their kidneys. That sick person is placed on a dizzying merry go-round.

Also destructive is the fact that the functions of the remaining organisms after their co-inhabitants have been treated is not acknowledged and so further imbalances almost inevitably follow... one after another after another!

Relinquishing Control to the Doctor

Another misjudgement in Modern Medicine is that of the practitioner, attempting to control the micro-organism but also controlling the patient. And the patient feels better because the doctor is in control. We have been programmed to relinquish our power and our innate intuition to the doctor. The urge for control, based on the need to dominate an enemy, is the significant issue.

The Bad Guy Myth

Related to the pursuit for the culprit disease organism, is the notion that the microorganism is the "bad guy." This labelling has consequences. Louis Pasteur was the most powerful influencer in placing the "disease organism" in the role of the "bad guy" in this otherwise wholesome film script of our lives.

Sadly, this fed into cultural driven beliefs that adversely affected well-being. To illustrate, one–common belief is surrounded in notions of guilt and punishment. This perspective is part of our modern culture when we blame ourselves for poor hygiene if an infection develops or for simply not caring for ourselves sufficiently. Maybe we toss blame on our diet or not getting enough sleep. Our thinking implies a direct causal effect.

Self-Blame

Self-judgment and blame has a negative impact, as I learned in my conversations with microorganisms and particularly with those implicated in disease. Discordant thinking exerts a pressure to the system causing a cascade of consequences which force the organism-towards the disease state.

Chapter 3: Aspects of Modern Medicine — Past and Present

Attacking All that is Not Us

An interesting older approach of traditional medicine is to spark the generalised response to things outside of the body. So, we aim to attack all of that stuff that is not us. As a strategy this can be far more successful than looking at specific disease organisms and deciding to kill them. However, it takes us back to a place where we are viewing the environment as something we need to control. And it also reinforces separation, the view of an enemy lurking at the gate.

Eliminating the Foreigners that We Don't Trust

Perhaps we consider that some of the microbes which we believe are serving us and rightfully belong in our gut, and this prompts us to really look after them. Maybe we will then take a probiotic or do a faecal transplant or some other direct treatment approach. What that means is that we consign the rest of the microflora – the others - to the role of organisms to eliminate, the foreigners we don't trust.

Ancestral Memories

A potentially useful approach is to look at the ancestral memories of the balance of micro-organisms. I refer here to how our microflora was balanced before the advent of modern agriculture, sanitation and medicine -- all of which have led to tremendous pressure on the microbes in our bodies.

Without question, sanitation and medicine have led to tremendous increases in our lifespan. However, they are also instrumental in the creation of tremendous stress in the microflora too.

So, looking at a past example of human microflora balances is not as helpful to us as we might have hoped, as this approach doesn't take into account the changes in today's world. There is no doubt that these microorganisms are in a state of rapid and massive change. We humans are glacial in comparison. We humans clearly need to make an adaptive shift.

Chapter 4: Modern Medicine Fails to Recognize the Role of Unconscious Behaviour

When I am referring to unconscious behaviours it is towards ourselves, fellow humans, plants, animals and microbes. Our current unconscious behaviour implies blindness and lacks any real perception of consequences. It's a type of tunnel vision blocking from view any needs other than our very own. These unconscious behaviours have some similarly unconscious manifestations, at least to the aware individual.

I outline several of these unconscious expressions and the consequences of these unconscious behaviours below. The list is only an illustration, and in reality, this summary could be extended into a book on its own.

Unconscious Behaviours

- **Bullying Behaviour**

Primarily, we treat our fellow humans, plants, animals and microbes with cruelty. When we bully, their needs don't come into play. Only our own. This one-sided strategy is never successful in the long term. Why? *Because bullying creates divisiveness and separation.* This is easily seen when we look at how this approach is applied to a segment of our society. Immediately we see the results of cruelty and bullying in the formation of groups of people who are extremely unlikely to integrate later into the general communities. The same thing is happening with our microorganisms, we have bullied them and cruelly excluded them from resources, and now we are surprised at how they behave.

- **Strong and Rigid Belief Systems**

In brief, strong and rigid belief systems-- along with their habits and patterns they create-- set the stage for disease.

We humans are so connected to purpose that we easily opine that there is a higher order involved in the changes in everything on the planet including changes in ourselves.

This higher order for an individual human might be the order coming from scientific rules. For others it might be a Divine order of one sort or another. It is observable that this matter of who has the right beliefs of what is the correct "order" is something we cling to and will fight for, almost more than any other cause.

As an example, it has been observed that there have been more people killed in the name of the "Prince of Peace" than for any other cause in the history of humans. All religions are capable of producing this totalitarian behaviour. And to this day we can see news reports showing this pattern of belief-driven behaviour all over the world and in all cultures.

This gross example of how a strong belief system can lead to grotesque behaviour is worth remembering when we consider this micro level conflict between our bodies and the microbial community inside our bodies. The reaction of the microbes to this crusade we humans are taking against them is clear and obvious. They adapt fast and this adaptation leads to greater and greater confusion as to the health status of the greater organism.

What is the effect of these frequent adaptations? What organs are functioning up to par and what are not? The state of our bodies today illustrates that our immune systems and the minds that look after this piece of physiology are totally unable to keep up with the diversity.

(See later Chapters on the five brains and also the ten mind aspects they each support. See also my book "Beyond the Ego.")

- **An Out of Balance Need for Control**

Originally, control emanated from the need to be creative. And here I am not referring to an artistic creativity, but the kind of inspired thinking that is able to solve societal problems. But today we have a massive increase in our powers to control. We are now at the level of monolithic control.

The control strategy is not succeeding in either our wider society nor in our relationship with our microbiome.

Consequences of Unconscious Behaviour in Modern Medicine

Every action, every single thought, every belief we hold - individually or collectively- impacts the environment in some way. And so, the global lack of recognition, acknowledgment, respect of minorities and those with less than or societally imposed lower status obviously produces deleterious effects. These negative elements are part of the strategies of Modern Medicine. In a sense, Modern Medicine is now archaic. We need to replace its principles with ones that fit the vastness of differing situations and conditions comprising our new world.   Then, a new creative setting can emerge and survive long term as a truly harmonious homeostasis.

NEGATIVE ASPECTS OF MODERN MEDICINE

- **Diversity is Excluded Rather than Embraced.**

The need for control in our contemporary cultures is fundamentally driven by fear, greed and is allied to the selfish need to exclude diversity. Once again, this strategy had some success over thousands of years. However, today the way for us to advance is to *embrace* diversity.

We can see that the exclusion of diversity permitted us the opportunity to monopolize resources which would otherwise be spread over diversity. This occurred strategically. We experienced the rise in agriculture and technology at the expense of the wider environment.

I freely acknowledge that without this greed driven strategy which led to mining and modern technology I wouldn't have the privilege to be sitting at my computer writing this book. However, the usefulness of this strategy is becoming more and more limited.

- **Violence is the Approach to Roque Organisms and Overpopulation**

We also need to revisit our understanding of rogue microorganisms and how they lead to disease. In the case of microorganisms such as Candida, the progression of disease works in this way. The disease usually starts on the skin, moves to the gut and the abdominal organs. It advances to joints, the heart and the brain and its neurological structure.

This specific type of progression becomes a factor in obesity, diabetes, and other metabolic disorders. But, extremely important to note is that this is not a migration of the Candida! The density of the populations of the Candida shift from place to place.

It increases in one place and declines in another, and so on. The energy of the collective or what I call "Hive-mind" moves but not the individual fungi. It is not a steady movement of the organism from location to location. It's more like a wave in the ocean.

In both cases - rogue organism and or overpopulation – the modern medicine approach is the same which is to kill the rogue organism or the specific microorganisms that have overpopulated.

(Message from the Candida – "If you fail to deliver perception combined with clear intention and purpose then there is no chance of harmony in the system.")

- **Modern Medicine, Diet and Consciousness... Causal Factors in Overpopulation**

The Candida always existed in the various tissues of the body. However, the ways in which the populations grow and decline in each location has shifted as they react to our medicinal, dietary and consciousness choices.

The perceived population movement of the micro-organisms is a response to our approaches to the organism. It's not the organisms that change, but the environment. During stress, for example, population density movement is inevitable if that stress is not regulated.

The definition of overpopulation needs re-examining as well. In homeostasis, populations are moving up and down continuously as the entire system responds to the presented situation. The prevailing opinion that there should be some imagined static balance point where each day there are only a few Candida in any one place is in contrast to true homeostasis.

PART TWO: Health or Disease, a Decision of the Candida and the Hive-Mind

Chapter Five: The Decision Involves Multiple Levels of the Conscious and Unconscious Minds

Candida were the first microbial Hive to work closely with me in my work with the Coherence Device. However, they weren't the first Hive I had worked with and I document others of these in my book "Earth Seeds."

The patterns of how Hives work, particularly microbial Hives, can be clearly seen in the Candida Hive. However, for ease of discussion we focus on Candida Hive hereafter.

Let's say we walk into a winter meeting at the office and notice someone sniffling with a head cold. As the person sneezes and the air in the room is filled with a fine aerosol mist carrying the viral capsules, we know instinctively that whether or not our body responds to this threat is dependent on our health in that moment. We know whether we feel strong or are weakened by disease, chronic stress or negative thoughts. In fact, we know whether we succumb to the disease in that moment we breath in the virus or whether we do not.

We literally make a choice whether to be aligned with health and balance or not in that moment! *And this decision emanates from multiple levels of consciousness including our unconscious.* The thoughts are then shared with the Hive-Mind. What is most important to remember is that when the information is clear and aligned with health, the Candida vote for a healthy balance and harmony. *Where there is great confusion and fear then the Candida vote more erratically.* And so, a lot of decisions are made on the level of the individual sub populations of Candida. But how is this data compiled into a decision? It is through the Hive-Mind.

The Candida Hive-Mind Organizes the Data from Individual Cells

I use the word "we" here rather than "I". The profound truth is there are many voices who vote based on information they are receiving about what a healthy state for this organism is like.

For example, if a patient develops certain types of cancer, it is sometimes assumed to be the result of the rapid-fire reproduction of Candida.

I hold an alternative point of view, and that is that the Candida in these cases is acting upon confusing data. It is as a result of setting up conditions where some cells in certain tissues become so corrupted that they are disconnected from the main system.

The cells may be dying so that the Candida easily digest them. This is the role of cleaning up these tissues. The cancer is a response to confusion. The Candida is doing its job by replicating rapidly but unfortunately based on faulty data coming from within.

From a western medical perspective, it may seem that the Candida are somehow hijacking the DNA replication processes within specific tissues, and the consequent creation of cancers result. Again, my view is that cells in certain tissues become so corrupted in their thinking that they are disconnected from the main system and possibly die. And this is largely because of misinformation.

Chapter Six: The Principles of the Hive-Mind Encourage Us to Thrive

In my conversations with the Candida Hive-Mind, I have observed and learned a great deal. And although there are many teachings of the Hive-Mind, I discovered that these four principles were a constant driver of the decision.

The Four Mandates of The Hive-Mind

- No Organism is our Enemy
- Each Organism has a role to play
- The Community needs to be in agreement.
- There is no need for control

These principles of the Hive-Mind. The way it behaves, both recognises our environment and also blends with it -- is changing second by second to one of more diversity and that it presents a way that allows us to thrive in this diversity and change. Such an approach would involve us in a process of learning from our microbial environment. And to hold certain with the knowledge that the microbial community is learning and adapting by watching us too.

Candida, the subject of this book is the uncrowned queen in the arena of adaptation and learning. It has been a great journey for me and my clients to begin to learn from it.

(Message from the Candida Hive-mind – "You say we shouldn't live in the joints or perhaps not in the brain or perhaps you don't like us living in the Liver. – We have always lived in these tissues. There is no tissue in the body where we don't live.")

Permaculture

We can look to agriculture as a parallel example. Here I am referring specifically to permaculture. Although postulated by different theorists in the early 20th century, permaculture was popularized in the 1970's. It's a naturalistic concept incorporating, amongst other elements, whole systems thinking.

This is obviously akin to treating the body as a whole organism. The alternate view we are presenting here in this book is one more closely related to permaculture, only now we are talking of the permaculture of the body,

Currently, in our general environment humans have steadfastly tried to eliminate one animal or to try to have only a very few crops or other food sources such as factory animal farms. If you drive through the wheat belt in Western Australia near where I live you will see this at a gross level. There are 12 million acres of wheat. Monoculture everywhere, and all other plant species sprayed to almost extinction. The animal kingdom is completely marginalised too.

In summary our need to control is out of all balance, both in medicine and the treatment of disease and also in our approach to growing crops. The micro-organisms are out of balance and the plant and animal kingdoms are also out of balance.

(Message from the Candida Hive-mind — "If you continue down the path you are now following of treating us as an enemy then the human is making a choice for suicide.")

PART THREE: A New Way of Healing... Conversations with the Candida

In Chapter Five, I raised the option of a new way of healing. This new way would recognize the rapid changes in our world and its diversity. And would involve learning from the microbial community. I received my first sense of their voice while working on the Five Brain Coherence Device (see description in appendices.) The conversations and the wisdom gathered from these dialogues have continued. It wasn't too long before I learned the Candida possess a consciousness, an innate intelligence far greater than we can imagine. I will explain more about this intelligence as we proceed.

As I mentioned in my introduction, the Hive-Mind exists without ranking. How then can such an entity like the Hive-Mind – without ranking -- cope with the human way of thinking that is so profoundly hierarchical? How can we bring them in sync with one another to create a new way of healing?

Chapter Seven: The Strategies of the New Way

In my research and during innumerable interviews with the Hive-mind of clients, I have uncovered six strategies that comprise this New Way of Healing which cannot operate unless the human and the Hive-Mind are in harmony.

1. Talk to the Candida

The first method used to bring the human and the Hive-mind into alignment with each other is to talk to the Candida. As an example, in my interviews with the Candida, I would ask why they were overgrowing in a certain area. Let's say that development occurs in the sheaths of nerve bundles as they enter the spinal column. The physiological effect here is highly disruptive to normal nervous system functioning.

I would ask them "why were they doing this?" The answer to this and any other similarly based question is to commence with bemusement. They don't get why the question is being asked. I would show them what natural functioning of the nervous system looks like and the way in which their actions were compromising this.

The light would come on. Always, their answer would include the current instructions on which they are operating. *The Hives intentions are based on what they are able to perceive from us, particularly what we are holding as intentions, along with powerful beliefs and feelings.*

The Hive has the capacity to borrow our emotions and intellect etc. This is dramatically increased as a choice for the Hive when you start talking with it. *It is hard to over emphasise this. It is a quantum leap of our understanding.*

2. Provide Accurate Information

Let's use liver cancer for in which the Candida was playing a role as an example. In this case, the Candida may well be reaching into the functioning of cell replication to manipulate the DNA of these target cells. If we ask the Candida what they are doing, they reply that they are assisting in the decomposition of these problem cells. They are helping to digest them so that these cells are no longer misbehaving. The communication of this need is coming from us. When shown what this means in the big picture with a dying human, the stock answer is: "the information they are given is faulty".

Over many conversations, I showed the Hive-mind the consequences of decisions it was making and acting upon. In each case they showed me how the information was coming from our minds. The situation was not their sole creation.

So here we have just covered two further aspects of the "new way." *The first is to actually talk with them. The second is to realise that they are working on information that is to them faulty.*

Indeed, the words I kept getting in the interviews were that the way communication is managed is "faulty." I heard this repetitively and consistently in these interviews with the Candida of any given client.

(Answers from the Candida Hive-mind – "We are a Hive and we know only to cooperate and to collaborate. There is no competition inside of our collective of fungi.")

3. Acknowledge that the Candida Hive-mind Operates Only in the Present Moment

This third aspect of the New Way, is that *the Hive-mind is completely in the present, there is no real place in their thinking for how we got to this present place and no place for where actions today will place us into the future.* My results with clients were much stronger once this was acknowledged.

The only previous time I had seen anything like this was in working with entities. Resolving tensions by using coercion of any kind around possession were completely hostile to all involved and just plain didn't work. The alternate was to recognise that the spirits had no concept of what we were talking about. The only way forward was to co-operate and collaborate. This topic is covered extensively in my book, "The Unseen."

4. Cooperate and Collaborate with the Hive-mind

(Answers from the Candida Hive-mind – "Our blueprint for action is to Cooperate and Collaborate. We take action based on collective need. We see all of your cells and the cells of the bacteria inside the body as being part of us. We attempt to cooperate and collaborate with all.")

So, we have the fourth aspect of the New Way. **We merely need to formulate ways to communicate. New ways of collaborating between our cells and the cells of the Hive for the purpose of improving the function of the entire system.**

5. Respect their Needs and Acknowledge Similarity to Our Own

What do these microorganisms and their Hive-mind expect from us? *Another important element is to respect their needs*. This requirement and others were provided by the Hive-mind in answer to my questions. As sentient beings we see the similarity of their needs to our own needs.

- **Kinship**

  First, a bit of background. When utilizing the Five Brain Coherence Device I am obviously working with five brains – the head brain, thoracic brain (or heart brain), gut brain, spinal brain, and the pelvic brain. Each brain is associated with a mind itself composed of multiple layers and other aspects.

  I will elaborate on this later on in the book, for now I will briefly discuss the emotional mind, associated with the thoracic brain (heart brain.) It operates on a few basic emotions like compassion, love, anger, fear, joy, etc.

  In finding common ground, I found that around the emotion of love, the Candida were able to identify with this when love is interpreted as comradeship. This kinship extends to other cells. All of the other basic emotions like courage, compassion and so on flow from these emotions and were experienced and interpreted by the Hive in one way or another.

- **Respect and Recognition of them as sentient beings**

  We need to see and respect their territory while simultaneously recognizing them as sentient beings. From a modern perspective we would see this as a non-violent way, particularly when they utilise my understanding of the work of Marshal Rosenberg whose seminal work is widely published. Even in my own earlier work using consciousness technique with disease organisms, the Candida responded that such techniques were violent.

6. The Last Aspect of the New Way is Non-Violence

(Message from the Hive-mind: "You act as though you are so high and we are so low. You treat us with disdain, acting as though you are all powerful. All such hierarchy is violent".)

According to the teachings of the Hive-Mind, all forms of hierarchy are violent. And why is that? Because silencing any voice requires the use of force, in some way. Conversely, in a non-violent approach every voice is heard. To understand a Hive, we need to get more understanding of how a truly non-hierarchical system works. **We need to learn non-violence.** Every voice needs to be heard. We need to get around the table with all of these microbes to understand more about the challenges each of us are facing.

(Message from the Hive-mind – "We know that you are single organism like a single cell, but that you are very complex. We are Hive – so are many all as one. You are one, made up of much complexity.")

Chapter 8: How Humans Are Like the Hive-Mind

The next step, after discussing how the Hive-Mind is similar to the human, is to explore how humans are like the Hive-Mind.

The potential for true coherence:

The Candida Hive-mind talks about cooperation and collaboration:

"We know *only* to cooperate and to collaborate. There is *no competition Inside our collective of fungi.*"

Clear intentions and information are of the highest importance. "If you fail by delivering perception without clear intention and purpose, there is no chance of harmony in the system."

"Our blueprint for action is to Cooperate and Collaborate.

We take action based on collective need. We see all of your cells and the cells of the bacteria inside the body as being part of our Hive. We attempt to cooperate and collaborate with all."

Every tissue in our bodies is able to think. Every tissue. This may be astounding information to some of you. The microflora is thinking at the cell level and the level of the Hive. Thinking also occurs across each of the five physical brains (biochemical processes) which are associated with the ten principal mind aspects. The subtle energy systems are also all thinking as well. When coherent, all minds and brains and tissues, subtle systems are in continuous and intimate communication.

Aggregating Data Like the Hive-Mind

The human has the ability process a large amount of data. This is especially the case in this digital age where information comes to us quickly and abundantly. And just like in the human Instinctive Mind, which is related to the gut brain, the Hive Mind in turn is making decisions on thousands of processes all at one time. And so, both our human Instinctive-mind and the Hive-mind are at ease doing parallel processes. This ability to process huge volumes of data is the same in the instinctive mind and the hive mind.

Creating Coherence by Honouring the Opinions of All

This is an example of how the Hive-Mind is more advanced in its thinking and need for resolution through a logical interchange of information than the typical consortium of humans. As described, the minds have many major facets and operate on many levels of consciousness. Each of these individual mind aspects is thinking continuously. These thoughts are necessarily sometimes in agreement and sometimes are not. It is vital for this to occur of course.

It is critical for one mind aspect to be able to question the thoughts and particularly the proposals of another. Most usefully is the harmonised or balanced case where some mind aspects propose something, others then question this, and others further work to reconcile the different perspectives. The way that comes closest to achieving coherence in this way is to be conscious of the input of all minds and all mind aspects. And to then give each mind a voice.

To achieve the most "Hive-like" situation we allow all of the mind aspects along with all other voices to be equal at the table. To humans this is seen as a very advanced form of "Coherence" and yet we can see that, this hard to imagine state for ourselves, is already easily achieved by the Hive. The desire to be right has been removed from the discussion. Every point of view is up for equal consideration. There is no bowing to higher authorities as there are none.

Operating as a Group

The ability to operate together as a group is another way for humans to be like the Hive-mind. This occurs in what I think of as a completely evolved matriarchal society in which there is no hierarchy. However, we can't escape the evidence that we humans by habit are hierarchical beings. And further, we have been programmed for eons to be patriarchal which means we have layers and layers of hierarchy.

Our job in the New Way is to only express the very natural aspects of this and to leave the shadow aspects of cruelty and manipulation far behind.

(Messages from the Candida Hive-mind – "For you humans to be more Hive-like you would need to wake up and come to the table. Your sleeping masses may look a bit like us but if you take a harder look, you will see the resemblance is only skin deep. They are just individuals who happen to behave in similar ways but all the while being asleep. They conform to their social rules and follow their leaders. On the other hand our hive is fully awake at all times. There are no rules for us, only data, perception, consideration and action")

PART FOUR: Consciousness as the Prime Modality in Healing

A Unique View of Consciousness and Its Application in Therapy

It is a persistent component of faith for many that everything is consciousness. This is expressed in various ways. For most, it's a tendency to be always looking for a divine principle in every aspect of our existence -- including the settings of the natural environment. This divine involvement is, for most people, a bit of the dark and a bit of the light. In fact, we tend to seek out the ways the dark or malignant divine aspect has an influence on the way we experience reality. But also, of course, we also look for the light or the so called, "God like" expression into our reality.

In this work, we are examining the way a single cell organism can be conscious. We examine how they group together with other single cell micro-organisms and from there to group with the cells, tissues and organs of our bodies. The subtle systems of our bodies are included. It's a story of allowing all aspects to be expressions of consciousness. And it's also a reminder to look for how the micro is creating the macro. This general approach says that the physical is an expression of the subtle. **A fundamental top-down view.**

This perspective differs completely from the western scientific view, fully developed over the past couple of centuries, where the view is that something which could be described as consciousness is seen as a product of mind level activity. Importantly it's created from the physical, so the view is that the physical creates consciousness. **This is fundamentally a bottom-up view.**

However, I base this book on neither of these dogmas, but rather on my direct observation. That observation was attained through working with thousands of clients. It is unequivocally held by me **that both views are equally true.** This of course is a troubling position for each of the two camps in this debate.

Western Scientific view is that the Physical creates the Subtle – **A bottom-up perspective.**

The Alternative or Philosophical and or Religious view is that the Subtle creates the Physical. – **A top-down perspective.**

My observation is that both are occurring at the same time.

(Message from Candida Hive-mind – "You mention there are over a million kinds of fungi on the earth, and over 200 of these are involved in disease in the human body. These numbers deceive. There are many more kinds of fungi in the body and we all are involved in some way or other with the physical processes of your body. If those processes are not optimal by your standards, then we each are playing a part.")

Taking this open approach, I can allow pretty much anything to be available and especially if the observations are therapeutically useful. My measure when I consider the approach to be valid or not is pragmatic. If it works and helps the patient heal, then I am most likely to use this approach.

The Placebo Effect and Beyond

The most offensive fact for modern allopathic medicine is the observation that if in therapy a patient believes a therapy works then about 35% of cases resolve themselves for no other reason. This is known as placebo and is the basis of the need for how double-blind therapy approaches are measured.

When I read about this statistic of Placebo almost 40 years ago, and I had recently learnt how to use hypnotherapy as a self-healing tool, and also to use it with others for many disease presentations, I thought to myself, all I need do with my hypnotherapy is increase the rate of placebo. By people just believing something would work, what if we could increase this 35% success to say 80% or more. I have fundamentally held this intention ever since. The invention of the Coherence Device came as a result of my explorations into Placebo.

Chapter 9: The Human Brains and their Multiple Minds

The Five Physical Brains

My view and the basis of my therapeutic approach is that we have five major physical brains, and that these brains support the functioning of multiple minds as well. This perspective is a modification of concepts by other thinkers and the dogma of several major schools of thought.

Head, Thoracic (Heart), Abdominal (Gut), Spinal and Pelvic Brains

The first two are the head brain and the brain of the thorax (chest). There is widely held support for their existence and functioning. The next quite commonly accepted brain is the gut brain. This has been supported by the scientific community while receiving significant support from many esoteric schools of thought too.

The last two major brains are the brain of the pelvis and the brain of the spine. The spinal brain refers to the whole spine and the afferent and deferent nerves that supply the Musculo skeletal system and also the smooth musculature and it is centred around

---

The Five Brains are physical structures located around the body. The *many minds and their aspects exist as non physical* consciousness.

Despite this, the Brains support the Minds and the Minds at the same time support the Brains. It is a two way street.

---

the sacrum. Science frequently views the Spinal brain as being a part of the Head brain.

For clarity, I should add that each specific brain contains neural ganglia and therefore is capable of thinking at this tissue level.

The pelvic brain is not commonly observed as a brain even though science recognises that there are significant neural ganglia (groups of thinking cells) in this area of the body. The neural ganglia can be found around the musculature of the pelvic floor, around and throughout the reproductive organs, and other pelvic organs like the bladder. Even though the pelvic brain is not widely viewed as a brain, I see it "functioning as a brain" commonly in the processes going on in patients and observe it to be critically important in the therapies I implement.

The first step in the therapeutic process is to establish relaxation between these brains. My Coherence Device assists with this and makes the brains more receptive to the intention of coherence between the brains.

Each Mind has a Yin and Yang Aspect

The Minds that these physical brains support are the various Intellectual, Emotional, Instinctive, Moving, and Relationship minds. In therapy, I find it useful to apply the principle of the Dao where we look at Yin and Yang aspects of these and very commonly this becomes a focus on the Masculine and Feminine.

I should point out that while these may appear to conceptually overlap with the Chakras and the Meridians and also the Nadis, these minds and brains are very different approaches to that taken by these energy systems. Indeed, in therapy we would reference the brains and the minds and then also these subtle energy systems as all being component aspects of the being.

Examples of how the Brain and Specific Minds Interpret information

There are few topics more annoying to a modern medical commentator than the effectiveness of subtle therapies like homeopathy and acupuncture. Why is that? The answer is that they have nothing in common with modern medicine other than that each approach has the intention to heal.

Modern Medicine is far from subtle. Its focus is on isolating a singular cause of disease, typically malfunctions in the large structures such as organs and glands. The physician takes charge and considers how s/he will help repair the body usually including the use of one or more pharmaceuticals each of which have side-effects. Although physicians vary in their approach, it is nevertheless aggressive and frequently the patient is overprescribed with medication. Antibiotics being the most notable example.

As an alternative when we are looking at Homeopathy, the physician starts from the premise that the body is a self-healing organism. The remedies themselves are most commonly created from naturally found sources of all kinds. Through potentization they arrive ready for the patient in creams or tablets – delivered in tiny doses to stimulate the healing process.

When a remedy is created there is a memory of the original compound, even if diluted many times to increase its potentization.

I should point out that the way I am describing things here is not the way a traditional or a modern homeopath would talk of them. This is my way of looking at this and so is purely my own interpretation.

We need to look for the ways these physical brains and also the minds can interpret this energetic memory footprint.

The brain most involved here is the gut brain which has many skills in interpreting substances. However, the mind most involved in managing the ways things are implemented is the relationship mind (associated with the pelvic brain) which has skills in managing communications between almost anything within the being.

Therefore, we have this memory of the substance along with the intention of both the creator of the remedy, and the client using it being interpreted by the mind (relationship mind). The relationship mind then takes action, based on its understanding of what to do to communicate these intentions to the various aspects of the being which then get to choose to take action or not.

In this you can see many places where decisions are being made, and hence many opportunities for things to become unstuck too.

Brain/Mind Process in Addressing a Health Issue

The following is a breakdown of how the body would interpret the memory of the substance and the intention of the maker and user of a homeopathic remedy.

The gut brain steps in as it is the most skilled in interpreting chemistry. This is true even for the memory of the substance and so we are talking about very subtle interpretation.

The relationship mind, which receives and transmits information, obtains the conclusion from the gut brain.

Simultaneously, it communicates the intent of the practitioner and of the client to various parts of the Being.

These various aspects of the Being choose to take action, or not.

If this seems a little confusing, I give a much broader explanation of the functioning of the five brains later when we cover coherence in more depth.

Chapter Ten: Different Schools of Medicine. Different Views of Consciousness.

Some ways that consciousness is viewed in traditional medicine are worth reviewing from this utilitarian perspective. Each traditional school of medicine views aspects of the body as though they are conscious in their own right. This view also creeps into the common usage of any language on the planet. In English we talk about "shouldering responsibility" or "having a gut feeling". In these examples the shoulders have the consciousness of responsibility and protection, and the gut oversees being instinctive.

This approach is widened in each tradition, so as an example in Traditional Chinese Medicine, the organs have very specific consciousness and also manage or promote subtle energy systems throughout the body. In TCM we have the example of a fully conscious part of the body, acting independently of say the head brain, to coordinate many aspects of functioning of the entire being.

How and why TCM works is perhaps to do with the extension of placebo, or perhaps these approaches may be in themselves accurately effective. Either way the techniques have utility and work for millions of people daily.

The natural extension of the concept is to consider smaller and smaller (or go the other way and then consider macro situations) aspects of both our own bodies and of organisms in the environment. In my work I happily consider the consciousness of everything from the planet earth,-the solar system and beyond and then down to a sub-atomic particle.

All evidence points to the Candida --and other microbes for that matter --receiving information from humans. Here we are talking on the micro level about the Candida interpreting the fluids surrounding the cells near to them. On a macro level, they are receiving information regarding such things as our belief systems and emotional states.

I'm not aware of many researchers considering this information flowing in the other-direction. On an empirical level it has been my experience that the Candida are extremely vocal. In my conversations with the Candida of both my own body and the bodies of other humans and a few animals too, I can report on the richness of information flow that is possible.

But how can this be possible? The short answer is that we can't yet scientifically explain how this operates. However, we can see the effects of the Candida's communication, so it is a simple step to consider this observation as though communication were in fact operating.

Whichever way you choose to handle this, whether a scientifically observable mechanism exists or not, let us focus on the ways in which the communication can be observed. And most importantly, exactly what sort of information is being shared.

(Message from the Candida Hive-mind – Your thoughts are our thoughts. The way you understand is the way we understand.)

Chapter Eleven: Risks in Receiving Information from the Candida Hive-mind

The information of the human is the information of the Candida. This seemingly beneficial fact also brings significant adverse potentials. The most important is the potential for extremely mixed information. And by mixed, I mean conflicting and contradictory data. And this also includes data that flows in parallel streams. Exponentially compounding this problem of overload is that a wide array of different intentions is added to this flood. Therefore, every situation brings mixed intentions, parallels, and conflict.

Can a System Based on a Boss, Work with a System Based on Equal Voices?

Humans are extremely structured with a definite boss and definite parts that follow. This structure or mode of operation is full of importance-weighting and directives. When you add this hierarchy of the human to the confusion of the differently motivated information, we can see that miniscule chances remain that a Hive-mind will readily and accurately use this information. To the Hive-mind, the information can only be perceived as chaotic. And so, the answer is " **they cannot work together without intervention."**

The Hive is accustomed to information, based on the observations of its single cell population, which are consistent and without conflict. It has almost no way to cope with purposefully misleading information and it takes everything it receives at face value. **The Hive can't understand or even recognise deceit at all.**

The Need for the Coherence Device is Evident

You can begin to understand the need for the Coherence Device to create a unified and consistent stream of data from the Hive-Mind. The device acts as a way of making collaboration a reality between the microorganisms and the human at all levels. It's a method to override the abundance of confusing and conflicting data.

Typically, when working clinically, my approach is "the more information, the client can access the better." However, in the case of working with Hive Minds our human complexity of thought in all of our minds as well as the tissues is a mixed blessing.

Chapter Twelve: The Consciousness of the Hive-Mind is the Model for Our New Approach to Healing.

As we delve into the way the Hive-mind operates, we can see a structure where every individual is responsible only for themselves and in that they are completely responsible. Further, because they are part of a Hive their individual responsibility always converts to a common direction being taken. They are not each responsible for each other but rather only for themselves. This response and its underlying motivation ensures that they cooperate and collaborate.

To be successful in communicating with the Candida around new common objectives we need to take this approach as well. We need to take one hundred percent responsibility for ourselves and then notice the commonality, the sense of unity which flows from this.

At face value this seems reasonable. However, achieving the preference of being plain and straight forward is a huge obstacle. We resist and struggle. We run masses of multi-threaded intentions and motivations-with complexities of these multi - threads coming from the multiple minds. This is what the Hive-mind needs to unravel and interpret in order to then be able to draw reasonable conclusions.

Chapter Thirteen: Complexity of_Interpreting the Minds and the Brains

In total, I work with five minds each of which is split into a yin and a yang. Further, each mind is split into four levels of consciousness all the way from the sub of the subconscious through the sub conscious and conscious, and all the way up to the super conscious.

Add to this are the five egoic components (which sit between the subconscious and conscious minds, and we have fifty mind aspects, each of which is processing their own intention and sometimes multiple intentions at one time. What I have identified here is just the tip of the iceberg.

Add to this is the thinking of each tissue which can also behave like a mind. It is a complete jumble to a Hive-mind!

The first and most critical work is to gain coherence between all of these motivations and aspects of the human. Second, we can acknowledge the complexity and show the Candida the accumulated evidence. From these two efforts, the Hive-mind will assemble the most consistent intentions, especially as they relate to physiological decisions within a tissue.

Chapter Fourteen: Motivations - What is Driving the Human and the Candida

All organisms simple or complex have a drive to thrive and reproduce. The more complex the organism the greater adaptability they have in the manipulation of their environment. The single cell organism such as an individual candida does have ways of interrogating the environment and indeed their motivation to communicate is common with a complex organism like a human.

At the level of the hive the picture changes. Now we are working with a complex mind, but one that is motivated in a different way to a complex single organism like a human. The motivations of the hive are to understand the environment better, so that the individual cells of its composition can therefore adapt to it better. Like the single cell the Hive wishes merely to thrive.

Humans vary further from other complex organisms such as a dog or lion in that the human has motivations around seeking surplus, whereas a dog or a lion seeks abundance. (See "Igniting Collective Will" for an in-depth discussion on this).

We can examine the impact of common human drivers. For example, it is a frequent occurrence for the human host to avoid being plain and straight forward with any other human or with any other being, and that the habit is rather to operate from selfishness, fear, or greed. When facing these lower consciousness motivations, the Candida simply cannot integrate the information.

Showing the Candida the way past these sorts of intentions is critical to success in therapy. Working with the coherence device at this level assists considerably.

PART FIVE: Consciousness and How We Can Work with Consciousness in Therapy

It is easiest to understand my consciousness driven approach through the case studies of real people I have treated in my practice. For many, I was their last effort in an agonizing search for a practitioner that could actually provide a cure.

Case Studies

Throughout the next part of the book I use case studies to emphasise points I am discussing. The first case study is integrated into this chapter, and the following chapters also have case studies however to keep the chapters uncluttered they are placed **in appendix 2**.

Case Study. Female. Middle Age. Personality Disorders, Depression and Anxiety

Particularly in complimentary medicine - after you factor in genital, mouth and gut overgrowths then Candida is next most often cited as being associated with psychological issues.

My practice sees many cases of both clinical and sub clinical psychological issues. There is an epidemic of depression and anxiety in our western culture and this is usually treated by common drugs under medical supervision. As a complement to such medical assistance, I have created a self-help protocol to address a cycle of mania, depression and anxiety.

Less talked about but also incredibly common in both clinical and sub clinical presentations are personality disorders.

If you are unfamiliar with these personality disorders then for general information, there is a very concise summary in Wikipedia.

Of particular interest to me in this case study are clear leanings toward several personality disorders without them being clinically recognised by a psychiatrist.

The traits of the client in the case study point towards borderline, paranoid, and schizoid. These are sub clinical in this case but are none the less disturbing for the client who also cycles around anxiety and depression.

To illustrate the management of depression, anxiety and mania, I have created a series of videos based on my experience. Easy to follow, full of healing tips, the series covers the general concepts in my approach and then the specific details of the method. There are 29 videos in the "Neil Dougan Depression challenge" and they can be found on YouTube Alternatively you can follow this link for video 5...A good place to start. https://youtu.be/rn3e5S5859k There are other

resources at www.neildougan.com as well.

For the client all of these personality issues lead to massively confused and multithreaded signalling from the various minds to the Candida and the Hive-mind which then weighs these various factors and determines action.

The paranoid tendency leads to a highly urgent sense that the Candida acts upon. Therefore, the responses of the Candida are highly amplified.

The borderline tends to conceal.

And the schizoid promotes highly compartmentalised instruction sets.

The anxiety and sense of helplessness (depressive) become reinforced too.

For our client in therapy this complex set of psychological tendencies has to be simplified for the Candida Hive-mind. Once this is done the dramatic physiological swings it has previously been supporting calm down.

Prior to intervention with the coherence device. The action of the Candida has been to amplify the physiological expressions of these psychological tendencies. These include: massive mood swings; digestive issues; respiratory issues; pain; mental confusion; lack of focus; increased fears and doubts, cyclical experience of sadness, and the compulsive urge to fearfully control everything inside themselves and in the environment.

Once the Candida has a clearer picture then the client also begins to see the dominant personalities more clearly. The client may for the first time remember how these are expressed across time periods and circumstances. The paranoia consequently drops with resultant reductions in the anxiety promoting pressure.

It is a complex set of issues for the client who with their newly improved communication and collaboration with the Candida Hive-Mind, begins to release the pain from everyday living. More joy and peace are now possible.

The Will of the Candida

The Candida Hive has a will but rather than being the will of a hierarchy it is the will based on a cumulative view of its environment. There is no single point of command.

If we think of a beehive, we assume that the queen must be in charge. But the reality is that there is no real evidence that she takes such a hierarchical role. Sure, the queen does different things within the Hive, but decisions appear to be far more democratic - based on the observable data and the weight of the consistency of that data.

The Hive-mind of the Candida is an even more flat arrangement. There are no queens nor are their specially adapted fungi. All single cell organisms are completely equal.

One way we can see an analogy in our world is a web of information such as the internet. Here there is just information. How we humans use this information is, of course, hierarchical. It is true we have the information from everywhere technically available, but we hierarchical beings have developed search engines and so on which effectively shut out access to most information. Therefore, as an example for us, the web itself has the potential to be reasonably flat.

For the Candida Hive-mind, the position from which action is taken is completely democratic. There is no posturing or attempts to persuade nor is manipulation possible for it.

We arrive back at the data coming from the human. It is a mess of contradictions and conflict.

Chaos in communication is the persistent outcome.

(Message from the Hive-mind — "Remember today you were working with Client x, and you asked us what was happening in a complex biological issue inside an organ, we showed you the conflict. Some of their cells were not perceiving the needs of some of their other cells, the first cells were deaf to the entreaty of the cells with the concerns. You asked us could we help, we said yes, you asked us what you needed to do, we said - join us and be clear about the intention.")

I used the term democracy before, however even this notion is misleading. The Hive operates on the weight of evidence, there is no proposer of a position who tries to convert the voters to their cause in opposition to the other side of a position. In clinic, I see this hierarchical approach time and again where one organ or system in the body or even down to subsets of these can set up a completely different position of need to another organ or system of the body. These then proposition other systems and organs for power or to find which will have the strongest influence.

As an example we commonly see that there is, in a chemically objective view, sufficient sugar available in the liver and blood stream for the needs of metabolism, and yet the appetite centres loudly tell the body that we need to eat an ice-cream.

The message from the liver is different to the message from the appetite centres. (Meanwhile the appetite centres are being completely held to ransom by our beliefs, memories, habits, and feelings – but that is a story for later!).

If we consider this situation, we can see this confusion in operation for the Candida. It is a common perception that the person's Candida gets involved in this and amplifies the appetite, making the decision to eat more sugars almost inevitable. The Candida meanwhile remains confused because the data it is hearing from the liver and blood is so contradictory to the dominant message from the appetite centres.

Here in our example we see the entry point for overgrowth. The Candida Hive portion that resides in the Liver and Blood decides it needs more information, so it increases the population of Candida in the Liver and Blood. We are creating this outcome due to the presence of the conflicting information.

This need for more data generally, and more consistent data in particular is one of the most persistent sources of the urge by the Hive to create Candida overgrowths.

My view is that the single cell Candida organism communicates directly to the Hive. So the message is standalone. The Hive organisms collectively note this information along with that coming from the billions of other Candida in the body. Where there is sufficient weight then the whole Hive begins to act based on this weight of information. The fact that the individual cells are living in wildly different circumstances is added to the confusion around action. It appears however that the desire for clean information is the main driver.

So, if the Candida is in touch with the minds of the human who - through the immune system -recognise the balances needed in microflora in any place in the body then how could an overgrowth be possible?

The answer is the conflict. The various minds are deluging the Candida with information and most of it is conflicting. The strongest and most persistent information and the need for clarity are what leads to the decision by the Candida Hive.

The Candida organisms directly perceive the environment through the chemistry they encounter, but for other data acquisition the Hive relies largely on borrowing the perception of the human.

Modern AI systems are similar in their need to acquire data, we can see some of how the Hive operates by looking at AI. The Hive has no subconscious aspects, all data is open, just like an AI. When the Hive encounters the subconscious elements of the human it has no way of differentiating it from the conscious thoughts.

The implications of this are far reaching. In therapy we endeavour to point this out to the Candida. Especially when the subconscious is so "at odds" with the conscious. If we label the thoughts of the

> The Candida Hive-mind has no way of recognising the difference between a subconscious thought and a conscious one. All thoughts are treated as equal. The need to gain coherence between the various subconscious and conscious minds is therefore clear.

conscious as priority weighting then the turn-around in the actions of the Candida begins.

Unlike a rogue AI of the Science Fiction world, the Hive knows when the balance it perceives based on the data it has at hand is achieved and it will not consume beyond that. Overgrowths are always, in my observation, based on the perception by the Candida that the level of consumption (what we term overgrowth) is actually appropriate.

Another example of how the conflict can lead to an inappropriate response can be seen with how cancer is created in the body. There is much research into how microbes can influence the creation of cancer cells and Candida in this role appears in much of this research.

My evidence is anecdotal after conversations with the Candida, but in my observation, Candida can indeed be a vector in the promotion of the tendency to create cancerous cells, but this promotion of the tendency only occurs after the weight of evidence to do so is large enough. Here the information is that the target cells are a problem, so they should be removed from the collective. That information however is often highly conflicted.

Parallel trends can also confuse the Candida. So here I mean that the parallels don't support each other but they also aren't directly in conflict. Here they are perceived to be robbing resources away from the other parallel. In these cases the Candida can attempt to limit this perceived parasitism around resources.

The information surrounding these parallel processes can be intermittent too, this lack of consistency is further confusing for the Hive.

For the opportunity for a human to collaborate with the Hive to go forward into a place of true symbiosis, there needs to be several things occur. Firstly, the contact between the Hive and our various minds needs to be respected and kept open as a priority.

Then we need to start listening, and make sure that we value the information we are receiving. Lastly, we need the intention to cooperate and collaborate to be clear. With that intention operating we put our resources behind the community understanding and decisions for action. With these things in place new vistas open for our health.

In a later chapter I will talk about how you the reader can work towards this outcome.

(Message from the Candida Hive-mind – "If you want to get cooperation with us then stop fighting us. Do what you can to avoid the urge to try to control us")

If we want to collaborate with the Candida we need to understand what the real strengths of the Candida are. The easiest way to introduce this is to recognise they are superb in all things to do with community, so our approach will be more successful if we limit our need for control and judgement, and to also allow the separation to dissolve away.

How would it feel if we threw away the need to control, and instead openly asked, "How can I help you today?"

To do this we need to work out a way of talking clearly to the Candida, and also to hear clearly what they have to say.

To illustrate this in a treatment setting I include a case study in the Appendix 2

Case Study 1 – Male middle aged, with lifelong intermittent Candida overgrowths in the groin area - appendix 2 –

This case is unique like all cases are -- but the principles can be widely interpreted. I will talk about self-help approaches in later chapters.

Chapter Fifteen: Suggestion: The Basis for All Therapies

All therapy is based on a suggestion to the body and minds. In the case of allopathic treatment, it is a chemical suggestion. It says to the body and or an aspect of the physiology, "Go on. Do this." This approach is somewhat like a sledgehammer at times, but undeniably successful very often. Many of the most common drug treatments today have results of 50 or 60%. And so, they come close to adding another 15 – 25% onto the placebo effect or just having the belief that it will work.

Complementary medicine also relies on making suggestions. We may choose to work with nutrients, diet, or with the subtle energies such as chi, kundalini, or the meridians. Maybe our approach includes the Pranic systems or the auras of the body. Perhaps we utilize intentions such as visualisations.

In each case a suggestion is being made. Homeopathy is particularly interesting case where there is a remedy where a carrier such as water is imbued through the potentization (multiple dilutions) with the energy or intention of the remedy substance.

My first training in Hypnotherapy directly applies here too. We make suggestions directly at the mind level even if we are targeting a physiological change.

I hold the belief that the subtle energy systems – chakras, meridians, nadis, auras, to name a few, -along with the minds form a higher aspect of consciousness with the spiritual components sitting above these,

The Placebo and Beyond

As mentioned before the most offensive thing for modern allopathic medicine is the observation that if a patient believes a therapy works, then about 35% of cases resolve themselves. This resolution occurs as a result of belief alone and is known as placebo.

How Suggestions Are Interpreted - The Five Brains and the Multiple Minds

In my view, which also forms an important basis of my therapy work, we have multiple physical brains, and that these physical brains support the functioning of minds of several kinds as well.

In the way I view things (which is a modification of the concepts proposed by many other thinkers I may add, to say nothing of the dogma of several major esoteric schools of thought as well) there are at least five major brains in the body.

The first two are the head brain and the brain of the thorax (chest). There is pretty widely held support for their existence and functioning. The next quite commonly agreed on brain is the gut brain. There is significant support for this from many schools of thought too, as well as from the scientific community.

The last two major brains are the brain of the pelvis and the brain of the spine (whole spine but centred around the Sacrum). The

Spinal brain is often thought of as a part of the Head brain in science. However, the last one, the Pelvic brain, is not commonly observed as a brain by scientific thought.

So, while it is scientifically recognised that there are neural ganglia (thinking cells) around the musculature of the pelvic floor, and also throughout the reproductive organs and other pelvic organs like the bladder, this is still not widely viewed as a brain, I however recognise its existence commonly and I observe it to be critically important in the therapies I am using. Ideally, this brain should work together with the others, easily. However, this is very often not the case due to conflicting and contradictory data and overload. My Coherence Invention approaches the way in which these five brains can become more relaxed and receptive to the intention of coherence between them all.

In therapy I find it useful to apply the principle of the Tao where we look at Yin and Yang aspects of these and very commonly this becomes a focus on the Masculine and Feminine. I should point out that while these have overlaps with the Chakras and the Meridians, and also the Nadis; these minds and brains are very different from these other approaches. Further, in therapy we would reference the brains and the minds, and these subtle energy systems as all being component aspects of the being.

In the example of homeopathy, where there is a memory of the chemical or other compound in the remedy remaining in the carrier (scientifically there is nothing remaining of the actual chemical after the remedy is sufficiently potentised), then we are looking for the way these physical brains and minds can interpret this.

The brain most involved here is the gut brain which has many skills in interpreting chemistry, however the mind most involved is the relationship centre which has skills in managing communications between almost anything within the being. Here we have this memory of the chemistry along with the intention of both the creator of the remedy, and the client using it, all being interpreted by the mind (relationship centre).

The relationship centre then takes action based on its understanding of what to do to communicate these intentions to the various aspects of the being. Then they choose to act or not you can see many places where decisions are being made, and hence many opportunities for things to become unstuck.

Expanding our knowledge to include these multiple minds and brains opens enormous opportunities for healing. I give a much broader explanation of the functioning of the five brains later when we cover coherence in more depth.

In the work we are discussing here we are looking at the way a single cell organism - a fungi - can be conscious. The consciousness of a single cell organism appears to us to be limited; however we can't really connect easily to all that is going on. The next giant leap by our perception is as these single cell organisms come together and the hive mind is born. Something far greater than the sum of the whole, an alchemic or quantum leap.

Our ability to connect at this level of organisation is generally sketchy, largely because of the human fascination with hierarchy as we have discussed in many places in this book. The magic of the elaboration of consciousness and the solutions and healing it brings continues as the various hives come together and head towards coherence between them all. Such coherence, perhaps through the grouping together with all of the other fungi of its type, then further as they group with all fungi of other types and then group with other microorganisms. (an example of microbial hives coming together is in Case Study 9)

For both the human and the Hive complex the next giant leap is when the fungi can then group with the cells of our bodies and then our tissues, organs, then with all of the subtle systems and so on. **It is a story of allowing all aspects to then be expressions of consciousness but also to look for how the micro is creating the macro.**

(Message from Candida Hive-mind – "You mention there are over a million kinds of fungi on the earth, and over 200 of these are involved in disease in the human body – These numbers deceive. There are many more kinds of fungi in the body and we all are involved in some way or other with the physical processes of your body. If those processes are not optimal by your standards then we suggest you observe that we are all playing a part in this.")

Case Study 3 – Female middle age - distressed sacral area with severe pain and some immobilisation. Musculature and the nerves associated with the striated muscles, their association with the joints including the bones, ligaments and tendons and muscles.

Case Study 4– Male Middle Aged - shoulder issue, with pain associated with movement and lack of range of movement. Non repair of shoulder injuries after an event of a fall some six months earlier.

Can and should current therapies be modified?

Given these new classes of observations of how consciousness arises, my belief is that current therapies would be of greater help to a patient if they were open to being modified. I have developed specific approaches which I can share in training with practitioners, but these are really outside the scope of this book. For you reading this chapter whether you are a practitioner of some modality or if you are an interested self-healer, then either way the new ideas presented here can be applied immediately.

- Allow yourself to "hear" the microbes in and on your body. Really suspend disbelief.
- Allow any ideas or images to come forth. Get comfortable with the fact that these communications are likely to be a combination of

    - information from an aspect of your subconscious

    - your desires and/or imagination, etc.

    - And all mixed in with the messages from the microbes.

- Be comfortable with this richness of communication.
- Measure the effectiveness and accuracy of the information over time
- Tune into the sensations that accompany reliable information and that of less reliable information.

By doing these things on a regular basis your perceptive ability to filter and sieve the flow of information will grow day by day.

Most importantly regularly ask for and set the intention for clear communication between all of these multiple arrangements of consciousness.

(Message from the Candida Hive-mind – "We are talking and talking and talking. Are you listening?")

Chapter Sixteen – How the Microbes react to our approach to them?

The reactions of Microbes to our attempts to control them is as diverse as the range of organisms, and more complicating also is also complicated by the as diversity of the range of what we are doing in our attempt to control them. In short, their response can be widely varying from moment to moment. This is the scenario all healers find themselves in right now. It makes tailored solutions for a particular microbe very inefficient, and a control strategy that is working one moment can be wildly inadequate the next.

The other side of this coin is how the microbes react when we try to cooperate with them. Obviously, this is the approach I am taking therapeutically, and the results are pretty interesting.

What we can see are some patterns. I speak here about the whole microbial community but with particular focus on the fungi and Candida Albicans in particular.

The very first work of this kind I did was with Viruses, I was particularly interested in the nature of a virus, and how that related to a consciousness.

A virus is basically a piece of simple genetic material usually DNA inside a capsule. The capsule serves to maintain an environment to protect the genetic material. It also has mechanisms both morphological and chemical to encourage potential host cells to allow it to come inside so that replication can occur.

From a consciousness perspective, aside from a bit of clever engineering in the design of the capsule, the virus is fundamentally information. A very clean form of consciousness.

I started to ask the question of this genetic held information – "What information do you bring to the host cell?" The answers were partially the expected ones about self-replication and so on, but most interestingly there was also information about general consciousness.

So information about how the host organism could better manage itself, based on what could be described as ideas for new designs for living.

To be clear here the virus has information to share about much better ways for a host organism to operate. In our case we are saying that the virus can be the teacher of the human. This approach is the focus of an upcoming book I'm writing on viruses, and this is the centre piece on my vision of the road to physical immortality.

More complex structures such as microbes including fungi expand on this trend. They bring messages of their own to the equation of communications. From what I observe the picture is even more amazing as these single cell organisms operate together in a Hive-mind.

When they are asked to share wisdom the results are amazing.

I consider myself a very lucky person and part of that good fortune or abundance is I get to speak with lots of Microbes as well as other forms of life.

Recently I was talking with a human about the lessons from the Candida Hive-mind. A persistent series of related questions from humans is "How can I make this happen? What do I need to do? What do I need to offer?"

For a human trying to get their head around how we can interact with microbes and for that matter how we can truly be communicating within ourselves, the issue first becomes, how can we operate in a way which is suitable for this communication? The answer always involves the suggestion to the human that they need to relinquish the need for control. To let go of the need to be in charge.

Flowing on from here the question of entanglement often gives us a nudge towards some kind of ownership stress. Ownership stress leads to either the restrictive feelings of duty and obligation, or, on the other swing, to the expression of the feelings of entitlement.

One thing the Candida Hive has taught me is another reality. One where everything is completely responsible for itself. A natural consequence of that complete responsibility is that we naturally take care of our environment as we recognise we aren't separate at all.

> The Candida have no contracts. They have no separation. They have no sense of hierarchy or ownership. If you wish to fully participate in their world you need merely give up all of those things. Just release them.

I remember at the beginning of my journey with this work. I was working with a human client who was suffering from severe digestive symptoms in which the Candida in her body was deeply involved. At the time being a hierarchical human, I was trying out a very human gambit with the Candida.

It was around food and other living conditions that they like. I said to the Candida – "If we give you lots of sugar to eat in other parts of the body will you then please reduce your numbers in the humans gut?". I was offering a contract to them. They were completely mystified by this bit of human thinking.

Habits, Beliefs, Emotions, Diet, Supplements as interpreted by the microbes.

Several of the case studies in appendix 2 show the kinds of direct responses that come from communication of the kind that could be described as one of "Habits", "Beliefs" or "Memories with an Emotional Charge". This concept of a charged memory/habit/belief is common in consciousness-based healing methods. These charged experiences have tremendous impacts on the health of the individual.

Our habits which give us a way of communication are also the very things that limits our success in trying to expand the success. Regardless, they are only the tip of the iceberg of how we are communicating with these microbes.

The next major way we communicate is with emotions themselves.

Many people are fearful of microbes, (not the warm fuzzy ones in the probiotics or yoghurt or other fermented foods, of course).

They can often feel hate towards them when they have a sore stomach, or itchy skin or a rash on their genitals or some unpleasant discharges etc. Other common emotions are those associated with feeling a victim, which would often include resentment or even sadness.

I observe in therapy that these emotions when directly associated with the disease presentation and therefore the microorganisms themselves are interpreted as direct communication with the organism.

> The emotions of the human are interpreted by the microorganisms as a direct communication. These emotions are complete and need no other thoughts to be associated with them.

Usually the organism assumes the feelings are their own feelings, but sometimes they can behave as though they themselves are victims of bullying, or perhaps being misunderstood and so on.

Another dominant way we communicate with the microbes is through *diet*. Here there is an attempt to railroad the microbes into a different pattern of behaviour.

The use of diet is therefore viewed as interference against the functioning of the Candida and or other microbes in their being able to carry out the common goals as they see them. The microbes view this as a form of violence against them.

Changes of diet inevitably attempt to starve one population allowing other populations to be more supported. This is further evidence to the Candida that their good work is being interfered with, and they are misunderstood.

Supplements fall into this category too but are also about encouraging some cells and not others. This can be viewed by the microorganisms as yet another form of violence.

Then there are drugs. Antifungals and antibiotics. These are viewed as just plain hostile, further a hostility to the self, as the Candida or other microbe doesn't really interpret separation. We are seeing the microorganisms viewing these drugs as an effort to damage ourselves, a kind of self-mutilation. Or perhaps even a suicidal intention.

Chapter Seventeen – Likes and Dislikes of Candida Albicans and many other Fungi.

When you are with your therapist and asking what to do about a fungal overgrowth, inevitably we find ourselves at this question. What is it that we are doing that encourages the fungi to overgrow?

If we are lucky in this scenario the practitioner will talk to us about stress in our life and the psychological responses to this stress. More likely though is that this question is immediately interpreted by the need to focus on the diet we are currently consuming that in turn best supports rapid multiplication.

All fungi and most bacteria consume sugars. We interpret this as sugary foods as being what encourages fungi. The bigger picture is far more complex.

All microbes including fungi have complex responses to other chemicals especially things that either stimulate or suppress. So all kinds of natural and allopathic remedies contribute here, as well as things, like nicotine, caffeine, cannabinoids and a whole range of recreational drugs such as amphetamines, cocaine, morphine, heroine and so on too.

The reality is that fungi scavenge whatever sugar-based food is available. This includes foods of many kinds, metabolic by-products, and parts of dead cells.

The later when looked at from the other direction comprises one of the profound gifts from the fungal community. They help clean up surplus "food like" waste material that is left floating about.

Without the type of consciousness intervention we are talking about in this book the cells of the body and the fungal cells get into a kind of nutritional tug of war where each is looking for access to more and more of certain nutritional components. Two of the commonly cited ones are Iron and Zinc, both of which are often in short supply so tending to define limits of cell growth.

It would then also be convenient to support this tug of war, but this approach is full of fishhooks too.

Another aspect of the environment convenient to fungi is lower oxygen levels, and also pretty acidic conditions. Again both of these are targets for nutritionists and doctors alike.

The cells of our body undeniably do better in a slightly alkaline setting and definitely are more comfortable with higher oxygen availability. So, if we are considering getting a more harmonious setting for the homeostasis, then we need to work with these natural tensions.

This is particularly important in disease presentations. The complications of Candida overgrowths aren't at all pleasant for the host and can lead to severe disease too.

So being mindful of how we can preserve safe populations is useful. The idea here is to work towards preserving safe populations for all organisms not just the warm fluffy ones in a probiotic☺.

Should we cooperate?

A completely different line of enquiry is to consider the likes and dislikes of the Candida on the topic of "should we cooperate with it or should we encourage a cold war between our cells and with the Candida?"

Now we are into territory which has no recognised specific science. So my comments come from a philosophical and intuitive perspective.

The first question that pops up is, are such questions even relevant to a single cell organism like Candida?

It seems that all life has a need to thrive, and to do so there needs to be adequate resources of all kinds, and that limiting factors to this thriving be minimised.

Given the chemical environment of a cell of our body in contact with a Candida cell, we are talking about conditions which may cause stress, and also factors of nutrient availability. In that way at this very basic level, enabling conditions where there are a lot of nutrients of all kinds available, and things aren't toxic then we are meeting the kind of conditions desired by each type of cell.

If there is a shortfall of resources we see another picture, one where some cells do better than others.

But does this philosophically mean that a certain cell type wants to deny another cell type? That competition is the only model?

Well, we don't know for sure, but my intuition tells me that this is plainly not true. My conversations with microbes make such a question seem almost ridiculous.

A bigger factor that follows is that we have such an incredibly diverse biota inside of us. Questions of bioavailability and toxicity versus limitations and constraint need to consider this complexity.

What flows on is that there are options for cooperation emerging all over. The cells of our body arranged as tissues, have specific needs which the microflora of our body can contribute towards as a natural part of their functioning. It isn't that we are asking them to do something difficult, it is all perfectly natural. Similarly, the needs of one type of microflora can naturally contribute conditions that support other types too. All without stressing the donor cell types.

In clinic it often presents that there is cooperation possible between viruses, and bacteria, and fungi all combined with one or more of our own cell types.

Interestingly this form of community which I think of as a Tetra is mirrored into the macro where I do come across opportunities to do work with a very different tetra, one composed of either two different kinds of entities, an animal and a human; or sometimes an entity, a plant (often a tree), an animal and the human. (See My book – "The Unseen")

There are no fundamental barriers to this kind of work, It is so useful to work with this form of collaborative structure.

There is no question however that the fungi, say Candida Albicans, absolutely love the stretch that comes from this collaboration. They get to observe the universe in new ways, via the other organisms involved. What this means is that in this question of what are the likes and dislikes of the Candida this is super important. They really like to expand their ability to interact with the environment, and if they can get the chance to share our perception and understanding then they will jump right in.

(Message from the Candida Hive-mind – "We communicate. Many Opportunities. We know and have regard for the viruses and the bacteria. You expand our possibilities. Thank you.")

Case Study 5 – Female Middle Aged – Ankle Injury not healing – See Appendix 2

Chapter Eighteen - Purpose, and the Information Field of Candida Albicans

All beings that exist in our perception field, from a virus up, have a corporeal, or physical aspect, and in some way or other also have sentience, and spiritual aspects, too.

Both the corporeal and the sentient have a purpose, and each of these interleaves with the other.

In the case of Candida Albicans and for Candida in general, we need to consider both a corporeal aspect and the sentient in both the form of the individual cell and in the form of the whole population, both inside the individual host and also within the wider populations or Hive.

So, let's start by looking at the single cell.

My view requires the concept of a divine principle to exist in all of reality, so we see it in a single cell organism expressed as both the individual and their personal climb to find their way back to the divine or as it is talked of a lot today "Source". This climb provides the impetus for change and adaptation. So, the population of individuals also have a perspective around self-perfection which inevitably includes the need for and all of the other makings of change.

This need for change expresses itself in the corporeal as an adaptation to the environment which includes genetic modifications to the DNA of the single cell. These genetic modifications lead to new strains of the organism that are ever better adapted to the changing environments. Important here is to remember that the environment is often trying to limit the success of these single celled organisms too. So they are finding change to cope with this pressure (generally competitive and often destructive in its intentions) as well.

So we have a picture of the corporeal single celled organism around the use of change as a strategy to succeed.

At the sentient level the single celled organism represents the divine in a pure questing nature to find itself. It is a sentience of perpetual self-perfection.

At this single cell level I observe the quest to adapt and learn to include the exploration of the possibility to cooperate with other cells of their own type, but critically also to cooperate with viruses and the cells of other types of organisms, such as other fungi, and bacteria, and incredibly, even to cooperate with the cells of the host as well. This is all happening at the level of a single cell.

When we move from the individual cell to the group of Candida Albicans at a single site within the body or even more impressively at the whole population level inside all of the various tissues of the body, we see this single celled pattern as a starting point and for this starting point to be wildly expanded upon.

At the corporeal level the opportunities to join together to manage stressors (remember the host and other organisms can either choose to be open to the organism, or completely hostile) is widely acted upon.

This leads to many of the conditions we consider to be disease for the host. So, in the case of the Candida, they collectively ensure localised lower oxygen level, more acidic conditions and so on. In short, they get the environment to suit their ease of existence wherever possible. This need to manage the environment requires communication leading to individual cells having coordinated action with each other.

For me, this pattern of behaviour (communication leading to individuals having coordinated action with each other) is viewed as the makings of both possibilities, one is for the group to side for only their own success, or alternately for the group to recognise a bigger opportunity at this corporeal level to cooperate with the wider environment.

So the opportunity for something wonderful exists inside of this same mechanism which can alternatively also lead to some form of disease or other for the host.

There are many ways that this can and does occur at the corporeal level. It is all in the way the chemistry surrounding the cells is managed.

Now we consider the super exciting possibilities of the sentient aspect of the Candida albicans as a group.

Here we have come into direct contact with the Candida Hive-mind.

While it was relatively common for me to receive information from the collective mind of many microorganisms, it wasn't till a client told me that the Candida actually spoke out aloud in his mind, that I thought the time had come to share my own experience more widely.

My early questions to the collective were about "what are your intentions?". The deeper questions around purpose flowed from those earlier conversations.

(Message from the Candida Hive-mind – We see you are a part of us and we are a part of you. We know this because of you. When we live in other animals it is different, there is not so much data, and the thoughts we share are different too.")

We see here that the Candida Hive-mind has a purpose and intention which echoes ours. The complication is that they are not organised in the same way as us, and as a result half of what they receive from us is jumbled at best, and often completely outside of their ability to assimilate.

So let us look at their organisation and see how that interferes with the communication of intentions.

As we have discussed humans (and most complex organisms in fact) are fundamentally hierarchical. There are command structures running in every direction. It does not mean there is one ultimate boss, far from it, but rather that something is always telling something else what to do.

Because of the complexity of having five minds associated with five brains and with each mind having a Yang and a Yin expression and for each of these 10 mind components also having a natural and a more egoic or imaginary aspect, and for the mind to have four levels of operation, things get complex to say the least. In the communication of intentions there are therefore multiple opportunities for confusion.

The Hive operates in a totally different way. It is completely flat in its structure. So we see a structure where there are not ever any bosses, nor are there ever any servants.

This probably sounds pretty awful as a form of government – how is there ever a decision and how does anything ever get done?

The answer is that all decisions on any subject and all held intentions and courses of current action are based on the weight of evidence. It is a very pure democratic form. Problem with using that word "democracy" is we immediately think of what we do in our so-called democracy, where we hand off responsibility to our government. We expect our elected leaders to be responsible.

So the Hive-mind is more easily seen as a form of pure anarchy. Every individual is completely responsible for themselves, and as a result because that responsibility includes the responsibility as a part of the whole Hive, their collective will naturally be coherent.

I have studied this in clients. In this real world setting there are populations in wildly different settings with very different biological processes going on. So we ask (well I asked anyway ☺) of the Candida say in the spinal column if they are part of decisions being made by the Candida in the small intestine. The answer invariably is that all decisions for all actions in all of the multiple tissues of the body are made by the whole collective. And these decisions are based completely on the weight of evidence.

I asked further about the issue that there were so many decisions being made all of the time. Do the local populations have more of a say? The answer here is that the local populations gather more of the information utilised in any decision but the decision is always weight of evidence based and made by the whole Hive-mind.

> This shows an important aspect of purpose for the Hive-mind. The Hive Mind exists purely to express the will of the collective.

This is very important, as we humans are very structured, so our work of interacting with the Candida can be focussed within the tissue where the interaction is occurring, our structure assists here, the weight of evidence held up for the Candida to see will therefore be concentrated and far more useful. The issue and challenge is how to express this in a way that is seen by the Candida Hive-mind as weight of evidence based, so information that is flat and uncoloured by any sense of any given aspect of ourselves being the owner of rightness and some other factor owning wrongness.

Case Study 6 – Male, middle-aged and wildly fluctuating between over-weight, and something that could be described as a more natural-weight. See Appendix 2

Chapter Nineteen – Common Candida overgrowth presentations.

Without the kind of work we are doing here, the universal story in all forms of treatment approaches is that at best Candida is an organism that we have to watch like a hawk, and control directly through our diet, hygiene, lifestyle, and through use of drugs.

To many this view is far too weak and Candida is the ultimate enemy.

My conversations put another story and philosophy into focus, however for balance this chapter talks about what is the usual human experience stemming from their interaction with Fungi in general and Candida in particular. Reading the summary below it is not surprising that what many people think is that "Candida is the Enemy".

The list of disease presentations is long and the tissues involve include much of our body, and I only mention the more common ones below. As you cast your eyes over this list observe, how so many facets of ill health can count, in some way or another, candida albicans as a contributor.

Skin and Mucous Membrane Presentations

Toenail and Fingernail – exceedingly common, here the fungi easily grows under the nail as well, and can seriously disrupt the functioning of the nails, the nails are often discoloured, mishappen, and can even fall off completely. Bacterial infections can also follow.

Oral Thrush – Often begins as flecks of white but can soon become a coating throughout the mouth and throat. Severe discomfort, often a particular smell and taste as well. If it continues it penetrates into the tissues of the mouth leading to other infectious activity as well.

Genital Thrush – Particular yeasty smelling growths leading to rash, and breakdown of the skin and even penetrating deeper into tissues. Often these growths will also spread inside of the reproductive structures.

Throat and Sinuses – Often an extension of oral thrush but sometimes completely standalone. The presentation is highly irritated membranes that are normally also weeping and sometimes ulcerated, usually white growths on the surface but often these exist well inside the tissue as well. If the vocal chords are affected then voice can be seriously impacted upon.

Ears – everything from the outer ear to the inner ear including auditory nervous systems can be affected. Hearing can be impacted upon in the cases where the growths are in the inner ear structures, and or in the eardrum structures including the small bones of the hearing mechanism.

Eyes – Growths in the tear ducts, around the back of the eye and rarely across the outside of the eye are highly uncomfortable. Where these are active near the nerve bundles exiting the eye there is a potential for the vision to be impacted upon. Not commonly talked about are growths inside the eyes themselves, these include retinal and the lens as well.

Nose – Similar to the throat and sinuses with the added aspects of the nervous systems working with smell.

Digestive presentations

Rectal – The rectal region has exposure to both the digestive environment and the wider environment of the skin. For this reason digestive growths can combine in intensity along with the skin growths around the groin in general and reproductive structures in particular. The result can be an incredibly intense irritation and often weeping sores will result.

Colon – The colon hosts a large portion of all of the microflora of the body (some 70 trillion organisms in all) The fungi as a subset are no exception. Of all of the microflora candida albicans is seen as wildly over-represented in the apparent imbalances in the colon. Growths In the colon are attributed to nutrition uptake imbalances, digestion failure, psychological disturbances, leaky gut and many more.

Small Intestine – Less talked about are overgrowths in the Small Intestine including the duodenum. Again these have major psychological impacts, as well as digestive functioning

Stomach. The contents of the stomach, don't suit the Candida perfecty as an environment so when we observe the candida in the area of the stomach it is usually in the walls and vasculature surrounding and containing the stomach. The ability to manufacture exocrine substances which would go into the stomach is a major factor impacted upon by these growths along with the musculature of the stomach (That goes for the small intestine and colon too of course)

Organs

Liver – The liver in it's excretive function is split between creating digestive enzymes, and endocrine or hormonal substances. This is added to an amazing diversity of other functions which include amongst the some 1000 functions metabolic and blood health. Any of the tissues involve in these 1000 or more functions can be caught up in Candida growths. The impact of these can stall or otherwise pervert natural functioning of any of these subset tissues completely.

Kidney – The kidney can see growths on both the blood side of the tissues, and also on the urinary side. The growths can occur on the nephritic tissues itself and as a result interfere with urine production as well.

Heart – The entire heart with all of it's components can host growths. They can even exist in the walls of the arteries and veins of the heart. The result of heart muscular growths is stress on the circulation.

Spleen – Often related to overgrowths in the blood, over growths in the spleen will reduce the management of blood purification a function which is shared with the liver.

Lungs – All aspects of the lungs along with the mesothelium which surrounds the lungs, and the pericardium which separates the lungs from the heart can host overgrowths. Lung functioning in general can be impacted upon, and the interrelationship between the heart and the lungs in particular.

Nervous System

Distal Nerves – growths can occur at either end of nerve routes. These growths impact upon both receipt of information into the nervous system, and also the transmission of data out to the tissues that effect change.

Entries to Central Nervous System – particularly alarming is the places where nerves enter and exit the spinal column where overgrowths can occur. There is potential for both partial and total interference with the functioning of these nerves. The structures which include the vertebrae and supporting musculature, and connective tissue can all be impacted as well.

Spinal cord – overgrowths here can selectively affect the communications between body parts or can affect all functioning.

Vagus Nerve – the other main route for nervous transmission other than the spinal column. The vagus nerve when overgrown loses capacity to communicate information throughout the thorax and abdomen, including all sensory data between all organs of the body.

Head Brain – Any structure in the head brain, or the whole of the head brain can become overgrown by candida.

Other Neurological Ganglia – not really considered in medical science, however vital in my experience is that effect of selective overgrowths on the neural ganglia of the four brains situated outside of the head. These overgrowths in my observation can effectively shut down the ganglia and hence the way that these would otherwise support the related minds. Here I refer to the support of the Instinctive Mind, Emotional Mind, Moving Mind and Relationship mind. Obviously, the Intellectual mind is impacted upon in the same way with growths within the head-brain too.

Psychological

The role of the microbiome generally in mediation of pretty much all neurological activity is becoming widely acknowledged. Matters such as depression and anxiety are two that have been comprehensively studied in science. Candida overgrowths in the gut nearly always affect mood in one way or another including outright psychological disturbance. Other areas of research emerging are the role of the biome generally and Candida in particular in the Autism spectrum as well.

The foregoing is a simplified version of the usual human way of viewing Candida Albicans. There are published scientific articles noting more seemingly positive roles taken by Candida within the body but they are far overshadowed by these negative experiences.

Chapter Twenty – Can we turn the equation on it's Head – What happens when we reach for Real Cooperation with Candida Albicans

Because we are so hierarchical in our very beings, the idea of releasing control (central to a hierarchy) to a microbe or even a grouping of microbes is almost impossible for us to really conceive. Almost worse is the idea of joining forces with a Hive-mind. It all just seems totally incompatible with our deepest, most strongly held, belief systems.

We can perhaps think about it as an intellectual idea or perhaps have warm feelings around being part of a team, but when it comes down to it, our very being – to begin with anyway – screams against this.

By reading this far in the book you will have already begun to relook at all of this and for many of you a new potential is strongly emerging.

The issue of us as a hierarchical being, and the Candida Albicans particularly when viewing the Hive-mind, being completely flat, means that we need to work to make the first steps towards coherence happening in the first place.

So to begin with what are the steps to reaching a coherent state between our being and the beings composing the microbial communities. It is actually a question that equally applies to how we relate to our wider environment, and also applies to how one part of our being relates to other parts of our being too, so it is well worth our while spending a bit of time understanding this.

I call this the 7 C's; Contact, Connection, Communication, Commonality, Cooperation, Collaboration, and finally Coherence.

So lets pull this apart a bit.

The first step is we need to make **Contact**. In one sense the Candida is chemically in contact with us all of the time, however we are attempting continually through our immune processes to break that chemical-based contact all of the time too. So, if we are looking at how we might turn the usual hostile relationship on its head, and go for a peaceful relationship, then we have to allow the Candida to remain in contact with us. This situation goes for further up the consciousness chain too. If our cells, their tissues, and our minds, feel uncomfortable with the nature and intention of the Candida as it is perceived, then we may want to intermittently have contact to know what is happening but we certainly don't want to maintain it.

If we manage to overcome our fear at many levels of the Candida, then we can try for some **Connection**. This is the process of maintaining contact even if the experience is a bit like touching a hot object, we all know the experience of picking up a hot cup, we just want to pull our hands away. To turn this around we need to have a higher goal which allows us to overcome our fear-based discomfit. To continue our metaphor, we can find a handle to the hot cup or use a glove.

Importantly here though the glove has to be one that still leaves us aware of the essential hotness of the cup, otherwise the connection and what follows isn't real. We have already seen in several of the foregoing case studies that the metaphoric cloth to hold the hot cup is always available to us, interestingly the other microbes often provide this bridging service.

Once we can maintain connection, then the **Communication** can flow. We have already got to a stage where the nature of the information is acknowledged and that we will persist in maintaining openness no matter what information begins to be shared.

Communication requires one party to speak and another to listen. When I began my work with Microbes, this was all in one direction, I was listening to what they had to say, but this was only the beginning.

What we do know is full open communication where everyone gets a say and everyone's voice is not only heard but is valued and it truly matters. For communication to operate there has to be a common language. Microbes don't have English as a first language so the language we share in must be something they can manage.

The reality is that like in the case of working professionally with people of different language bases there are ways to translate things. It is a bit different for different kinds of microbes, but in the case of the Candida they sequester the systems of the minds, so they can communicate in an incredibly diverse set of ways.

I just think my communications to them, with focus and intention to communicate. They reply using thoughts, feelings, perceptions and pretty much all other kinds of ways that I would normally process thinking.

Now things get interesting. We are sharing data and intentions; we have the opportunity to disagree with each other or alternatively to decide on a common way forward. Where there is potential for a common way forward then we work to assemble those things that contribute to **Commonality**. To go further we need to agree to accentuate what we have in common, understand what we do not share, and decide on the balance of things what to do.

In working with Microbes, things like the disease expression of their activities are not agreed upon, whereas the common goals of everybody growing, and evolving and thriving are more of an open opportunity.

Cooperation which follows here refers to each party doing what it can to further the objectives of the other, as well as what parts they can play in an overall objective goal. In the work with the Candida, it is immediately obvious where all of the strengths and weaknesses, lie, and the Candida is always willing to do those things they are best at. As a practitioner it is a matter of highlighting the parts all can play, including all of the parts of the host, then sitting back and watching the cooperation occur.

With the processes of cooperation in regular practice we can then go for **Collaboration**.

This refers to outcomes that are well beyond the realms of the individuals even to achieve their own contribution to such an outcome. An example here with Candida is that they are completely flat in their structure, when collaboration kicks in they can potentially borrow the understanding of such things as dualities and hierarchy, which are so central to a joint project with many issues for a human.

For me as a practitioner it has been a complete revelation to experience how a totally flat structure performs, every aspect of the collective completely responsible for themselves, and so therefore no competition, a complete commonality in intention. I could only experience this by entering into collaboration with the Candida of both my own body and the bodies of Clients too.

> The Hive has the capacity to borrow our emotions and intellect etc. This capacity is dramatically increased as a choice for the Hive when you start talking with it. The choice is further accentuated when you are offering to collaborate. It is hard to over emphasise this.
>
> Collaboration is another quantum leap.

Lastly, we have the opportunity for **Coherence** to arise. A place of complete peace and harmony between all beings within us, and for it to exist between all aspects of the Human as well. This along with the relationship of the human to the wider environment. As practitioner I often get to observe this as a destination for my client or for myself.

Full coherence across all of our brains, and minds and with our microbiome and beyond is something we can get tastes of right now and move towards in it's fullest expression as we progress on our journeys.

Case Study 7 – Male Senior. Viral infection. – See appendix 2

Chapter Twenty one - How to renew and reprogram your relationship with the Candida Albicans in your body.

For many babies one of their first experiences of disease is a Candida infection around the genitals, or sometimes in the mouth. So we can't say for many people that there has ever been a particularly good relationship between the Human and the Candida.

The fact that Candida is present in almost every tissue of the body and has the potential in any of these tissues to grow to large numbers, and in the process then altering the background chemistry significantly making the normal physiology of the body exceedingly difficult, is another cause for concern for most of us too.

The intention of this book is to replace the normal hostile response to this capacity and nature of the Candida, with a response that recognises the needs of both the Candida and also of the Human.

The case studies in this book show this approach in operation from a practitioner perspective. I'm not suggesting a reader can just read this and then instantly be able to have no issues with the Candida of their body – It takes work. However, any reader of this book can learn how to do this type of self-treatment work and if you are already a healer then the approach that I am taking in my work can be learned too. The more practice you get, the better and more accurate will be the outcomes for you.

For practitioners of a huge range of modalities, there is much in this approach that can be applied. If you are interested, I have videos on YouTube talking about how some modalities can easily add this work into what they do. You are also welcome to reach out to me directly via email or through the website.

To prepare for conversations with your own Candida, you will need to begin with the mind state that will allow this. I include all of the 50+ mind aspects in this, indeed for the next steps in heading to coherence with the microbiome I need to explain more about coherence and the five brain, ten mind model.

Five Brains – 50+ Mind aspects – Natural Coherence, and added help from the Coherence Device

I grew up in a school of esoteric knowledge which had at its roots many strands of wisdom including religions and philosophy. Esoteric here means that we were taught how to see the inner meaning within life and also within the various dogmas we come into contact with.

One philosopher from the early part of last century who had a huge influence on the creation of a modern understanding of these ideas was G.I. Gurdjieff. There are many books written by and about him and those teachings.

The esoteric drive to find balance is extremely common in all teachings.

I have taken these ideas and looked for ways to apply them directly in therapy. One strand of thought that prompted the multi brain approach was that sitting underneath the western religions, it can be seen in Cabalistic teachings, as well as in Sufic ones too. The origins of this thought are in the mists of time and include Persia, Egypt and the Eastern and Western Mediterranean traditions. They can be found elsewhere too.

The five brains refer to places in the body where there are large concentrations of Neural Ganglia. These are the Head, the Thorax (Chest including the organs and other tissues), the Abdomen (including the organs and other tissues), The Pelvic Area (including the organs and other tissues), and the whole of the Spine (centred on the Sacrum and Coccyx, importantly these neural ganglia are centred in areas of concentration outside of the spinal column as well as within it)

To be fair and for clarity I should mention that the traditional esoteric gnostic schools tend to group the Spine, Pelvis, and Abdominal brains into one overarching structure, but they do separate the mind aspects to a certain extent.

I have however found it extremely useful to separate these locations of neurological concentration into separate brains. So my definition is created to make the therapy work more simple, it is therefore a decision based on utility. This Five Brained approach with the Five Brains and Ten Minds in four levels of consciousness plus the egoic is thus a significantly novel adaptation.

Each of the physical brains is exceptionally important to the operation of the physiology of the body. Good and well trusted communication between them is an absolute must for optimal health. They can communicate via the nervous system, the endocrine system, as well as via the various circulation systems. They also communicate via the subtle energy systems, such as Chakras, Meridians, Kundalini, Pranic, Subtle Bodies etc, etc. In short, the physical can communicate in many ways, and when we encourage all of this communication to be truly open, trustworthy and complete this forms an important aspect of our self-work and is absolutely vital to the therapy work too.

To make this a bit easier to visualise I have made the following simplified table. It represents the most basic and commonly useful aspects for therapy which are the five brains and the major mind elements of the subconscious and conscious.

To this is added the Sub of the Sub-Conscious, a place where the subconscious itself can't look into, and the Superconscious which sits above the conscious mind, and reaches out into the universe. And lastly the Egoic level, to create a more complete picture. This wider picture is certainly useful in therapy on many occasions.

This latter layer of the ego is a big subject and vitally important in working with long-standing chronic and acute diseases, including all psychological issues as well. For more detail see my book "Beyond the Ego".

Simplified Table showing the Ten Minds with their five different levels or aspects, and their Relationship to the Five Physical Brains		
Head Brain	Yin Intellectual -sub of subconscious -Subconscious -Egoic (Deluder) - Conscious - Superconscious	Yang Intellectual -sub of subconscious -Subconscious -Egoic (Deluder) - Conscious - Superconscious
Thoracic Brain	Yin Emotional Centre -sub of subconscious -Subconscious -Egoic (Distractor) - Conscious - Superconscious	Yang Emotional Centre -sub of subconscious -Subconscious -Egoic (Distractor) - Conscious - Superconscious
Abdominal Brain	Yin Instinctive -sub of subconscious -Subconscious -Egoic (Denier) - Conscious - Superconscious	Yang Instinctive -sub of subconscious -Subconscious -Egoic (Denier) - Conscious - Superconscious
Pelvic Brain	Yin Relationship -sub of subconscious -Subconscious -Egoic (Separator) - Conscious - Superconscious	Yang Relationship -sub of subconscious -Subconscious -Egoic (Separator) - Conscious - Superconscious
Spinal Brain	Yin Moving -sub of subconscious -Subconscious -Egoic (Controller) - Conscious - Superconscious	Yang Moving -sub of subconscious -Subconscious -Egoic (Controller) - Conscious - Superconscious

Each Brain has associated with it a Mind made up of two parts, a Yin and a Yang. These are each also split into five mind aspects.

The Coherence Device in it's current version 3 can address all of these and many of them all at one time if that is therapeutically sensible.

The two parts we are covering here are a Yin aspect, and a Yang aspect. When they are balanced they form a single functioning Mind component. However they are so often imbalanced that it is a useful therapeutic and extremely valuable self-development approach to see them as separate aspects that each need to be worked on in order to bring about that balance. In addition to balance with their own counterpart in the mind it must also be in that state of balance with the other minds. Convenient as it may be to think of these two mind aspects merely as being masculine and feminine, there are many other ways in which duality expresses itself.

The mind associated with the head brain, is the Intellectual mind or Intellectual Centre. The mind associated with the Thoracic brain, is the Emotional Mind or Emotional Centre. The mind associated with the Abdominal Brain is the Instinctive Mind, or Instinctive Centre. The mind associated with the Pelvic Brain, is the Relationship Mind or Relationship centre. And lastly the mind associated with the Spinal Brain is the Moving Mind or Moving Centre.

As I say, each of these has a Yin and a Yang aspect, and they are so often not similarly capable, and complicating matters further so often they are at odds with each other. So as a consequence it becomes easier to treat them separately. So as an example I may refer, say, to the Yin subconscious Intellectual Mind.

These minds have aspects of themselves within each other too, so as an example there are Yin aspects of the Moving Mind part of the Emotional Mind. We can go to this level of detail in therapy if it is necessary for this level of precision. Certainly in the self development work it is extremely useful to be able to gain deep understanding of what is driving you at any moment and to be able to make changes accordingly.

Another way of considering Ego is to recognise it as being closely aligned to the conscious mind. However it reaches for data from all of the mind aspects. You could also split the conscious mind into a natural and an "ego like" part in therapy as well.

I have YouTube videos and training on how all of this can be applied in therapy. These Egoic components are briefly summarised below. As mentioned before for full details see the book "Beyond the Ego"

Intellectual Mind	Deluder – The imaginary idea we hold of ourselves. This is the construction of our conscious mind intellect that is so often involved in disease, and includes how we weight memories, and our beliefs
Emotional Mind	Distractor – Our so-called negative emotions. These are how we usually intersect with our environment and also cloud our perceptions of all kinds.

Instinctive Mind	Denier – All of the confused patterns of instinctive behaviour, which come as a result of the confusion in information coming to the instinctive centre from the other minds and the environment. The end result is being certain about everything regardless of the origins of decisions. Usually to the complete exclusion of any other explanation.
Relationship Mind	Separator – The urge to disengage from the environment, and the urge of one aspect of our being, to separate from another or others too.
Moving Mind	Controller – behaviours around making sure the environment meets our expectations, note that many of these expectations themselves are resulting from the thinking of these shadow aspects of the conscious minds.

The esoteric self-development work of these various traditions is to exercise each of these minds to the point where they become fully functional, and, at the same time, to dramatically improve their interactions with each other.

The traditions I grew up around particularly suggested that all of life should be based around a type of balance where three of these five brains, always including the Intellect and the Emotions, where involved in all decisions. The format in this "Balanced" approach is that one Mind would Initiate, another would Question this initiated approach, and the third mind would work with the other two to Reconcile the varied positions of the first two. Thus it is commonly talked of that we make Three-Brained or Three Minded decisions. G I Gurdjieff a Sufi Teacher called this approach the Fourth Way, or the way of balance. Generally, this is approached while leading an everyday life.

I have referred here to the western approach, however this approach is exactly mirrored in the Eastern approach of Taoism too. If you scratch the surface of the dogma a bit you can find it in all other major world religions and in all other Eastern schools as well.

In therapy we are suggesting the same thing only now it is expanded out to the entire, brain/mind system.

As they say everything is vibration and resonance is achievable through matching vibrations. To me this is most easily accessed in therapy through suggestions of some kind when we are talking of working directly with mind activity.

I had worked with Hypnotherapy since I was an adolescent. I recognised later in life that the hypnotherapy mainly targeted the Intellect with some influence over the other minds too, but definitely most strongly focussed on the Intellect. I observed that a therapy like homeopathy targeted the Instinctive mind as a first priority. It is a set of chemical suggestions of a very refined type. And so if we have the time we can look at all of the healing modalities and see how they suggest predominantly to one mind or another, often via the physical brains too.

The suggestion aspects of the therapies are interpreted and used by each layer of each of the minds, however it is in the subconscious of each mind that the action occurs most obviously. It is for this reason that V2 of the coherence machine used the frequencies suited to the relaxation and alignment of the subconscious. Of course the Conscious Mind is always involved too as so much of our understanding resides at that level.

How I got started with the frequencies to promote coherence.

In my journey that led to the research around the Coherence Machine, I had developed a range of subliminal affirmations for various health applications, and I noticed that these were of course, gaining only partial traction with the minds other than the intellect.

I used a very common technique to encourage the physical head brain into a more relaxed and hence receptive state, one where the physical brain doesn't, get in the way of good mind activity. The relaxed and receptive physical head brain wave state is called Alpha and is an important component of all meditation approaches. So I used the common technique of binaural beating, to encourage alpha into the head brain, and like so many other practitioners, I too achieved good success.

The new developments of the various coherence devices followed on from this. I started with experimenting with ways that I could encourage all of the Five Physical Brains into a relaxed and receptive state too. I tried many different ways to do this all based on the use of frequencies applied as best I could directly into the neural tissues.

The early results of the experiments asked as many questions as they answered, however I eventually settled on the use of the four new frequencies, tailored to each of the other four physical brains. (I continued working with alpha for the head brain of course.)

I successfully tried using pulsed sound, electrical, magnetic, and electromagnetic emissions of various frequencies directly upon these physical brains, but finally settled in the end for using pulsed non-visible light of a frequency that will penetrate the body into enough of the neural tissue to potentially stimulate the physical brains to relax and become more receptive. This is a far more accurate mode, but all of the others I tried worked to some extent or other.

This pulsed non-visible light approach has proven the most successful so far.

The obvious extension of this Version 1 approach was to look for frequencies for each of the sub-conscious minds which I finally was able to identify., I built these into version 2 of the machine, to assist not only the physical brains to relax and become receptive, but also for the subconscious minds to do the same too.

Version 3 which I later completed also applies this approach to the remaining parts (the conscious, sub of the subconscious and the superconscious as well as the egoic)

It was through the use of the version 2 machine that led me to a new more open dialogue with the microbes, they literally opened up a dialogue with me as I lay on the machine myself. At the time I was doing some treatment for a client I was working with at a distance. It was then that a dialogue with the microbes stepped up a gear.

It is far from essential to have one of these coherence machines to get started though.

The knowledge of the experience of this coherence working for me is enough to assist you in becoming sufficiently coherent to allow a communication to begin to be established with say your microbes, and with Candida in particular.

Getting started with Conversations.

So lets go back a few steps to a place you can begin from. My own journey to get comfortable was to first get comfortable with accessing information from the subconscious aspects of each of the five minds.

The easiest way I know to achieve a growing successful experience of this is to use any one of the dowsing techniques. In any of these a question is asked, a silence is held following this and then the answer is presented. I have a video showing an extremely easy to learn approach to this using a pendulum, freely available on YouTube.

A bit of a spoiler alert here - Expect to be presented with false leads and other "white noise" in the learning of this process. I have shown thousands of people how to use a pendulum and the experience of false leads appears to be a bit unavoidable. But my reassurance to you in the face of this is that along with the expression of patience your success will come.

To help with the false leads and other white noise I show in the videos ways to allow for the cross checking of the answers you are getting. Once you get comfortable with this, then the false leads can become useful in themselves, as the false leads are often stemming from other information trying to make its way into your conscious minds.

Be aware that each of the ten minds has it's own conscious and its own subconscious aspects (along with superconscious and sub of the subconscious) so the information we are retrieving using the pendulum can be coming from any of the 10 subconscious minds. (Both a Yin and a Yang aspect of each of the five minds). A later step is to open up the dialogue with the deeper sub of subconscious, and superconscious and then to general consciousness.

Remember also that the answers you get from the pendulum will be the answers held true by your subconscious. They aren't supposed to be some kind of objective truth, but rather useful information for how you are creating your own reality from within your own subconscious.

The answers from the subconscious mind aspects are the "held-truths" of the particular subconscious mind aspect which answer. And the answer will be dependent on which of the five subconscious aspects have answered. They are not some kind of "objective truth".

So practice, practice, practice.

Once you are comfortable with drawing information from your subconscious minds, you can start working with other information sources. One that is available to anyone is information from the earth. The techniques are similar, but the intention is different. After that you can try other information sources such as parts of your own body. Again you can ask a question of any body part using the pendulum. You can check and cross check all of this.

Lastly you can ask questions of something not truly a part of you, such as say the Candida.

The first thing to be aware of here is that you are now asking questions of another being which has it's own agenda, and, comes complete with its own varied experience of you.

I had to practice for a long time and with the eventual use of my Coherence device which helped as well before such communication with the microbes all started falling easily into place.

Once you get comfortable with this dowsing and or muscle testing approach you can start using a more meditative approach, which is what I do now with all clients. To be clear though, I definitely started with muscle checking and other dowsing techniques like the pendulum first.

Now I merely enter a meditative state and pose the questions or offer the suggestions in my conscious mind and then all of the communication at all of the appropriate levels occurs. Further the information is shared up and down in the layers of each mind from the sub of the subconscious all the way to the superconscious.

I took the steps I mention above to reach this point. All it takes is patience and practice.

So we get to the question of how to gain a better relationship with the Candida (and other microbes too) using some additional aspects of these approaches that you can apply right now, and of course if you are interested in doing training in these techniques then look out for the links at the end of the book and videos mentioning training, or get on an email list or join the Facebook group too.

If you are serious about following this line of approach, then access to a Coherence Device will accelerate your success. The coherence machines are under productions now so look out for them along with the training I provide.

OK so you have developed the capacity to actually receive information from the Candida (or many other beings too of course).

What about them receiving information from you?

Well don't stress about this, they are aware of everything going on in all of your minds already. They can't necessarily make sense of what you are saying, but they are definitely receiving the raw information. Of course, the huge complication for open communication is that in the normal human condition the information that is flowing is so conflicting from one mind to another.

So why would we bother even trying given we humans are just so full of conflicts and parallel motivations. Is it all too hard? Well if we don't bother and make the change to open up real dialogue then we remain in the battle with the microbes in our body and also with the ones in the outer environment too.

For me there was no other real option that made sense, I just had to develop ways to clarify and simplify my messaging to the Candida and to other microbes.

Again we see the Candida are only following the best options as they see them. – Because this statement is seemingly so unlikely, - we ask again. Why do the Candida believe that they are doing the "Right Thing"? And - How could they be getting it so wrong?

The critical thing is to understand the needs of the Candida and other microbes and why they are making the decisions they are. Also to understand what information our system is providing to them to lead them to the belief that they are doing the right thing.

The thing the Candida and the Hive-mind in particular want above all else is clarity. Remember they assemble matters based on the weight of evidence. What we need to do is get the important stuff in front of them in such a way so they recognise it as being really "Weighty"

My approach is to set up a protocol for communication which clearly shows the kinds of mind information which I intend as really important to the Candida and the Candida Hive-mind. To use a metaphor I'm waving a flag, jumping up and down, and shouting out "This stuff is really important".

(My message to the Candida Hive-mind – "When I parade the structure of my brains and minds before you, then the next messages and questions I send are very Weighty, they outweigh other messages you are receiving from me, and are the highest priority".)

My technique included showing the complexity of the ten mind, five brain model directly to the Candida via the Candida Hive-mind. I showed how it is possible for a human to have one line of thinking happening in one mind and completely different ones occurring in the others. I showed that some of our minds can be having many thoughts all at once, meaning that potentially there are hundreds of thoughts occurring all at once.

For you to get a better more urgent and weighty line of information going to the Hive-mind you will need to do this too. I have YouTube videos demonstrating this, some of which are guided meditation style videos you can listen to as you do the meditations. I also have a range of audio meditations on the website which will help.

Another way that would assist here is to use any one of the several techniques developed by the Heart Math Institute, these have many components but the ones I'm thinking of as I write this include a Heart focus, use of gratitude and use of the breath.

The result of such practice will be on the path to what I am terming five brain coherence. I strongly recommend looking into their work which as I say has well proven results for coherence between the head brain and the thoracic brain. My clients who are familiar with these techniques report that they are then more easily able to also start down the road to full "Five Brain Coherence".

So one way or another get yourself into Alpha through meditation, and bring awareness to all of your five physical brains, then slowly bring focus on the ten minds with all of their aspects too, setting up as much coherence as you can in all of them.

Set the clear intention to communicate with the Candida.

Then parade through your conscious mind, the structure of the brains and minds. For most of you this will be a visual or idea based parade or some combination of both. Allow time for this parade of structure to be completely clear inside the intellect.

Breath this complete awareness of the structure into each of the other brains and the minds, one at a time. Sense how each mind has a slightly different way of interpreting and then expressing this structure. Allow each brain and mind time to become fully engaged and as coherent as possible. Assemble this diversity that each mind is sharing, and parade all of it through each of the minds one at a time.

Give a clear suggestion to the Candida and the Candida Hive-mind, that this parade of structure will precede all weighty communications from you to them.

Once you feel that this has been achieved, which for many people will take several meditations to obtain, then confirm through dowsing that the message has reached the Candida and the Candida Hive-mind. Be kind with yourself and allow whatever time scale is needed. Go back as often as you need. If you feel you are getting stuck seek out the various videos and so on available on the website etc detailing each step.

Once confident the parade is reaching the Candida as a "Weighty Message", take yourself back into alpha and commence the communications. Do the parade, so the Candida know the information following is weighty. They will then know what to do.

Introduce what you would like to see occurring. Always express gratitude to them for the opportunity to collaborate with them, allow love and compassion for all beings, including yourself, to permeate your ten minds, feel it in your body too.

The communication will now have commenced. The confusion will begin to dissipate. The Candida will understand what you would like to be happening.

They will begin telling you of what they and the rest of the microbial community need. What their experience has been up till now. And what is motivating them. They will share the main areas of confusion around what your core intentions are. You will be able to work with these conflicts and come back to them with a more coherent message. One with even more weight.

Case Study 8 – Male – issues with creating abundance – See appendix 2

Chapter Twenty Two: The Way Forward

Thank you for reading this book. I am grateful to you.

The way we view and treat our fellow humans is mirrored in the way we view and treat our microbial community in our bodies.

Our news reports are full of the threat our neighbours pose. We are limited into a cause and effect cycle which permits only a very small range of outcomes. Generally we see this is around a lack of trust with feelings of fear and righteous anger following on.

My suggestion to you is to work to change this in this micro region of your life. Find a way to collaborate with your microbes. Find common intentions. Have gratitude for the roles they play.

My experience with my clients is that when they begin to make changes in this micro scale, that huge changes follow on in their wider world. In their relationships and especially in their relationship with themselves.

At the beginning of this book I spoke about placebo which is the effect that belief plays in healing. I said about my adolescent self, reading about placebo and wishing for a way we could increase the number of cases where clients became well as a result of intention and belief.

All consciousness techniques are working with this goal in mind, it is not unique to this work. However these new tools lift the game significantly.

A huge component of success is the extent to which focus can be applied to this healing intention and of course for the intention to be focussed in the right way.

With the development of this coherence work we have a new more powerful way of applying focus not only from our head or perhaps from our heart. Now we can purposefully activate all brains and minds to apply them to the healing intention.

You can do this too.

Appendices

Appendix 1:
Coherence Device

The Coherence Machine I mention in this book started as a question I had long harboured. Is it possible to hypnotise all of the five brains? My experience was that this process of relaxing the neural tissues, and coordinating them which we term hypnosis, was possible for the head brain and for the thoracic brain too. I had seen yogis who appeared to have hypnotised their pelvic brains, but that technique was not one I could use myself, and certainly not in therapy.

In any case I wanted a technique which could easily be applied.

My Trim programme which utilises binaural beating to assist the head brain into a relaxed Alpha state was the beginning. I took the idea and extended it into the rest of the brains. So now we work to relax these five physical brains. We begin to observe new levels where matter is responding to energy.

This encouragement to relax through frequency I refer to as entrainment.

Soon after the original physical brain work I felt it might be possible to also entrain the minds into a more relaxed state. Again I had seen and also personally experienced deeply relaxed states in several of the minds too, however it was always via a meditation of one sort or another. And this is almost impossible for the average person to achieve for all of the minds at once. (Hard enough to maintain one or two minds at once in reality.)

I was most interested in entraining the subconscious aspects of each of the minds. So this focus was built into Version 2

So even as I created versions 1 and 2 of the Coherence Device, with the ongoing trials it was clearly indicated that a version 3 was viable.

Version three expands the 10 mind aspects work out further to include the other three major aspects of the minds (Sub-of-the-sub-conscious, Conscious and Super-conscious added to the Sub-conscious), in both a Yin and a Yang aspect. Also it was clear that the shadowy or imaginary aspect of each of the conscious minds (which we call Ego) should also be entrained. So now we are working with 10 mind aspects for each of the five physical brains, as well as the five physical brains too, so 55 Human frequencies in all needed for this aspect of the coherence work. In some cases we also harmonise the Yin and Yang aspects and use an averaged frequency. This brings the total to 80 Frequencies. In clinical work so far subsets of these are applied. Usually they are applied directly to the Brain location involved, but sometimes also the frequencies associated with one brain are used on another brain too. (This is the case in the Candida example I post later)

Lastly the Candida Hive-mind itself has a natural relaxed frequency, so that is added into the mix too.

I keep asking the Candida Hive-mind if there are frequencies needed for the minds of other microbes. They have been enigmatic so far ☺ That may well be the subject of another book!

Many other frequencies have subsequently been added into the list of useful approaches these include manifestation, and the work with the unseen beings (subject of a later book)

V4 of the coherence device is now in small production lots, It has 200 independent light sources to stimulate neural ganglia and is programmable from a mobile device. For more information reach out to me.

By buying this book or contributing via Patreon you are assisting me to continue this research so thankyou again.

Chart of basic frequencies for the Coherence Device

	Physical Brain	Sub of Subconscious		Subconscious		Conscious		Imaginary/ Egoic		Super-conscious	
Head	9	53	49 Yin	796	792 Yin	1324	1320 Yin	1241	1237 Yin	1823	1819 Yin
			58 Yang		801 Yang		1329 Yang		1246 Yang		1828 Yang
Thorax	19	86	77 Yin	601	592 Yin	1418	1409 Yin	1272	1263 Yin	2129	2120 Yin
			96 Yang		611 Yang		1428 Yang		1282 Yang		2139 Yang
Spine	28	71	57 Yin	946	932 Yin	1331	1317 Yin	1295	1281 Yin	1931	1917 Yin
			85 Yang		960 Yang		1345 Yang		1309 Yang		1945 Yang
Abdomen	6	45	42 Yin	415	412 Yin	1214	1211 Yin	1019	1016 Yin	1728	1725 Yin
			48 Yang		418 Yang		1217 Yang		1022 Yang		1731 Yang
Pelvis	92	235	189 Yin	573	527 Yin	1558	1512 Yin	1469	1423 Yin	2616	2570 Yin
			281 Yang		619 Yang		1604 Yang		1515 Yang		2662 Yang
Candida	Hive-mind 4212										
Non-Physical	962										

Candida Healing Work – Coherence Machine Settings

The frequencies below are a good starting point, but are widely supplemented in therapy

	Frequencies Used
Head	796 (Subconscious Intellect); 9 (Head Brain)
Thorax	601 (Subconscious Emotions); 19 (Thoracic Brain)
Abdomen	415 (Subconscious Instinctive); 6 (Abdominal Brain); 1241 (Ego); 1272 (Pain Body); 1331 (Controller); 1019 (Denier); 1469 (Separator); 4212 (Candida Hive-mind)
Pelvis	573 (Subconscious Relationship centre); 92 (Pelvic Brain)
Spine	946 (Subconscious Moving Centre); 28 (Spinal Brain)

Text for Audio to assist in activating the cooperation and collaboration between Human and Candida Hive-mind

The full Parade of My being meditation text

- I am, I am here, I choose to connect. It is my purpose to evolve, I choose change which allows me on the path to peace and perfection.
- I am the Deluder. Even though my ideas have kept me from the thoughts of the Intellect, I love and accept myself as I am. I now choose to merge my thoughts to match the thoughts held by the Intellect
- I am the Distractor. Even though my feelings have drawn me away from the feelings of the Emotional Centre. I love and accept myself as I am. I now choose to merge my feelings with the feelings of the Emotional Centre
- I am the Denier. Even though my choices around the processes of the body lead me away from coherent physiology, I love and accept myself as I am. I now choose to merge my interaction with the operations of the body, to mirror the Coherent actions of the Instinctive Centre.
- I am the Separator. Even though I resist contact, connection, communication, cooperation and collaboration, I love and accept myself as I am. I now choose to merge my thinking and actions with the natural thinking and actions of the Relationship centre. I now choose to be open to coherent interaction with my

Environment. Each day I say to the universe „I am Here, I am available and I am ready and I desire to connect".

- I am the controller. Even though I resist the flow of creative options that change would bring, I love and accept myself as I am. I now choose to take action to support myself. By supporting myself, I also support others in their journeys too. I now choose to merge my thinking and actions with the natural thinking and actions of the Moving Centre.
- In the ever present here and the eternal now, I evolve and I grow.
- In the ever present here and the eternal now, I am responsible for myself.
- In the ever present here and the eternal now, I choose to hear and respect the needs of the microbial community.
- In the ever present here and the eternal now, I recognise and act upon the creative opportunities that include the coherent interaction with the microbial community
- In the ever present here and the eternal now, I show openly to the Candida Hive-mind, and the Microbial Community my five minds including the Sub of the subconscious, subconscious, conscious, egoic, and superconscious aspects

Video Resources

Dowsing
Basic Introduction to using a pendulum to get information from the Unconscious (Part of the Series on Geopathic and Environmental Stress)

https://youtu.be/mHpEqlay4CM

Consciousness Layers
What are the layers of Consciousness Introduction - https://youtu.be/BRR5gjEx_B0

Sub of the Sub Conscious - https://youtu.be/CKlRTb_OfQ0

Sub Concsious - https://youtu.be/wWb1FzxP198

Conscious - https://youtu.be/maPA4kHN7Bo

SuperConscious - https://youtu.be/68wdttLnocw

General Consciousness - https://youtu.be/8UJPdBLAabl

Five Brain Model
What are the Five Brains - Introduction to this modification to the Gnostic approach - https://youtu.be/cofUGRJEJnQ

Head Brain - https://youtu.be/CciurR4Neck

Thoracic Brain - https://youtu.be/Mol9Bu9FKa0

Spine Brain - https://youtu.be/xjEjcl_F2Dg

Abdominal Brain - https://youtu.be/3faNXoG0pf8

Pelvic Brain - https://youtu.be/hLOVJf41WRE

What is the difference between a Brain and a Mind? https://youtu.be/LYmUaJMOQvU

Five Minds and the Yin and Yang aspects
What are the Five Minds

Intellectual Centre/Mind

Emotional Centre/Mind

Moving Centre/Mind

Relationship Centre/Mind

Instinctive Centre/Mind

Imaginary or Ego Mind Levels

Introduction to the Egoic (or some people think of it as the shadow) levels of the minds. - https://youtu.be/IT8ZIU1BNYM

Deluder (Aspect of the Intellectual Centre)

Distractor (Aspect of the Emotional Centre)

Authority (Aspect of the Instinctive Centre)

Separator (Aspect of the Relationship centre)

Controller (Aspect of the Moving Centre)

Making sense of the 50 mind aspects and five brains.
Combining Brain with Mind and with Consciousness Level and with the Yin and Yang aspects – Introduction

Self Help tool to navigate to answers from all of the mind aspects (You can use this tool over and over)

Practitioner Series
Under development - See details of upcoming resources at www.Neildougan.com

Training Options

Training is dependent on whether you are already a practitioner and so perhaps wanting to add this knowledge and techniques to your practice, or if you are starting off and want to help yourself and your family and or perhaps to develop a practice yourself.

You can do all of this work without a Coherence Device. Having and using one regularly just makes things more accessible far faster. The purchase of a coherence device comes with detailed training on its use and how to gain the cooperation of the microbes in both yours and your clients bodies as well as for many other applications of course.

Particular focusses are also on the more subtle aspects of psychological issues including, Anxiety, Depression, Mania, Personality disorders of all kinds, the entire Autism Spectrum, and all Learning Delays.

If you aren't getting your own coherence device we have many other training options specific to the work with microbes. This includes mastermind groups and one on one training. If you want details of how that could help you go to. Www.neildougan.com

Link to Depression - Anxiety Cycle Videos - http://neildougan.com/change-the-game-depression-challenge/ - twenty nine of thirty videos in this series can be found on one page there. My own story which is episode 5 is here - https://youtu.be/rn3e5S5859k

The obvious question of where is video 30 is answered that I haven't made it yet as it is in reality going to be split into at least another 20 videos 😊

Guided Meditation to gain the cooperation of the Candida Hive-mind and other microbes -

Parading Structure to improve the weighting of your suggestions with Candida Hive-mind

The text version of this is below

The audio meditation is at www.neildougan.com

Breathing regularly and fully into the whole of the lungs, filling out the diaphragm with each in breath, then as you breath out allow the diagram to relax fully and then with gentle contractions of the abdominal and chest muscles allow all of the breath to flow out.

Breathing in and out steadily. Allow all of the five minds to relax with every breath.

Breathing naturally, allow an awareness of the thoughts of the head to come into focus, see their activity from the outside view. Just observe them in their action with every breath. From this observer place feel the peace and silence that exists in your intellect

Now focusing on bringing the breath to the Thoracic Brain focusing on the heart, feel the connection between the Head and the Thorax. Allow the thoughts of the Intellect and Ego to naturally subside in favour of the connection between the head and the heart. Watch as this connection grows, and the busy mind retreats naturally in your focus. Allow the experience of love to come into your focus, the love which reaches from the microscopic inside of yourself, out via love of self, and further out to your wider environment. Feel this Love swell in your heart.

Breathe now from the heart and the head into the gut, breathing down into the whole of the Abdominal Brain. Bring the focus of this breathing to the feeling of Coordination. Breathe the experience of a perfection of being from the Head and the Heart into the Abdominal Brain and feel it surge back to the Thorax, and to the Head as you feel the natural experience of everything in your being joining in with the perfect rhythm of life. Observe the Denier and the Pain Body and the Ego in operation, see how they tend to intercept this flow whenever there is disease. Allow the love and peace to join the coordination in the Abdominal brain and feel the interference to the operation of the Abdominal Brain subsiding.

Continue to breathe the peace, and the love and the coordination.

Bring your focus now to the Pelvic Brain. Sense your pelvic structures, and reproductive organs. Breathe now from the Head and the Thorax and the Gut into the Pelvis, feel the connection that is offered.

As you breathe, feel the gentle massaging of the pelvic floor as it too participates in every breath.

With each breath sense the natural urge to connect fully within your system, feel the waves of peace and love and coordination, flowing into the pelvis and respond from the Pelvic Brain with waves of connection and community. Focus on these feelings of warmth and community. Observe the Separator in its tendencies and watch how it urges disconnection. Watch as this urge is comforted and lessened by the community experience flowing from the Head and the Heart, and the Gut.

Breathe now from the Head and the Heart, and the Gut, and the Pelvis into the spine, focussing on the sacral area. Feel the peace, and the love and the coordination, and the community, flow into the spinal brain. Become aware of the Spine and it's urge to take action and to collaborate with all of the other brains. Be aware of the impulses of the Controller. See how the Controller tends to lead to hierarchy and violence within you. As you continue to breathe in the Peace, and the Love, and the Coordination, and the Community into the Spinal brain, observe the urge to control dissipating. With every breath feel the flow of action and taking responsibility flooding back to the Pelvis, to the Gut, to the Heart, and to the Head.

Continue to breathe into all five Brains, feel the coherence between them emerging.

As you breathe become aware of the Minds associated with each brain, sense into the Intellect, and into the Emotions, and into the Instinct, and into the Sexual, and into the moving.

Recognise with every breath that each mind is composed of multiple levels, feel the purpose of this design, feel gratitude throughout your system for it.

Breathe into the sense of the Sub of the Subconscious, knowing that information here is being allowed to synchronise safely with the information in the other minds.

Breathe into the Sub-Conscious levels. Feel gratitude for the free flow of information from these processes into your conscious mind.

Breathe Into the egoic levels, be aware of their circular patterns of thought. Be aware that they are the imaginary constructs of the conscious minds. Feel the urge for them to increasingly match your conscious mind, feel this process with every breath.

Breathe into the conscious minds. Feel the natural capacity swell in the Intellectual, Emotional, Instinctual, Sexual, and Moving Centre Minds. Sense their connection to the Subconscious and Sub of the Subconscious.

Breathe into the Superconscious level of all five minds. Observe the connection from here to the infinite. Feel the abundance of flow from here back to the other mind levels. See the support that is endlessly flowing from the universe.

As you breathe observe the Yin and the Yang expression of each of these mind levels. Sense the opportunity for harmony and balance, and for the opportunity for this duality to go back to its source which is unity.

Continue to breathe and feel this awareness growing within this meditation that here we have the observation of the parade of our being, and feel the growing sense that this parade joins our spirit, and to that of the divine, and to that of our guides which together compose our entire being.

Repeat three times. "This is the Parade of my Being".

Breathe freely now, allow the awareness of the oneness inside of your parade of being

Open this parade now to the microbes that make up your inner environment. Including to the Candida Hive-mind, and to all of the trillions of corporeal and sentient beings that share your body.

Repeat three times. "I am here. In this parade you can know my intentions to cooperate and collaborate with you. My intentions are clear, I have the will for perfection within my body, and minds, I seek your support in achieving this goal".

Continue Breathing and as you do so allow the natural abundance to flow, including the open information flow between the microbes and yourself, and also between all of the many aspects of yourself.

Appendix 2:

Case Studies

Note to Case studies. I wrote the draft of this book at the beginning of 2020. This was the concurrent with the beginning of the Corona experience.

The content for the book was in large part based on a slice of the sessions I was providing to clients at that time, with definite references also to my lifetime of work and personal discovery as well.

There is therefore a strong relationship between the case study and the content of the particular chapter it relates to.

Important - The last Case study (9) was written over a year later in June 2021, it is a very different case study and points to many issues only briefly touched upon in the balance of the book. The Candida Hive of this client asked for this work.

The content and purpose of Case 9 is therefore that of the Hive.

Case Study 1 – Male middle aged, with lifelong intermittent Candida overgrowths in the groin area.

There are no other obvious overgrowths around other parts of the client's body. Outbreaks are intermittent, and treatment has been through the topical application of antifungals of various types.

Other treatment has been to work with consciousness and diet. Flareups are also sometimes occurring within a few days of a sexual encounter, but, more often than not, they aren't associated with sexual activity either.

I treated this person cognisant of the approaches we have been discussing above. For this case study I show the dialogue between me as practitioner and the Candida of the client, with references to the client as well.

{"I am the practitioner Neil, my intention is to help resolve issues for Client x, in such a way as to ensure that every one's needs are recognised. Client x has the experience that there is an overgrowth of your cells in the area of the groin and particularly troubling to the client around the foreskin, this causes him pain and other discomfit, including psychological distress. Do you have anything you wish to show us or to say to us about this or any other matter?"

The Hive replies "We are aware of the seasons (at the time of the interview it is high temperature West Australian summer). We see his core temperature is a bit high too, but really the core temperature isn't so much of an issue, it is the temperature outside of the body and the change in humidity that we are experiencing right now."

I continue "Are you referring to the local temperature, and humidity of X's skin in this area?

"No. We speak of the temperature and humidity of the general environment, it is so hot and the moisture around is so low. We sense the fungi all around us, in the soil, and around the plants and trees. We know this is the time of urgent action."

"You speak of the seasons and your awareness, however you often overgrow as the client perceives it at other times of the year"

"Yes but this is what we observe right now. There are other reasons when we grow say in the winter"

"Are you aware of this seasonal information from the minds of the X or are you getting this information directly from other sources.?"

"We hear this information from many sources, but the loudest voices are the fungi living in the soil and around the plants near to X"

"Are all Fungi in the body more active when the environment is hot?"

"No. We are just more aware of these things. It is also a factor of how we work"

"Is there some way that X or myself can reassure you that you don't need to react in this way to the information from other fungi, can we show you that there is always plenty of moisture for you, that there is no scarcity in the body of water, nor is there ever serious lack of the heat that you need to help you to grow?"

"Yes, talk to us, we need strong consistent information that there is always sufficient moisture on the skin where we are growing."
–

At this stage I as practitioner highlighted the way temperature is managed in the body, the high water content of the body, how moisture migrates out to the skin even when it is cold. I showed it how it could access X's Intellect on this topic, and also X's

Instinctive centre (another mind managing much of the physiology) to gain further clarity, I also showed the moving centre of X (another mind) and how it understood the physics of chemical gradients and the way moisture was moved. Lastly, I also showed the high weighting of this information. They already knew that there was always plenty to eat, we covered this too.

"Are there other issues involved in this growth around the groin? I can show you the damage to X's body and what that means for him and his body?"

The Hive replied - "There is specific information which I can share about the location of our growth. There is much confusion about intentions in this part of X's body. We base this on what we perceive from the minds of X, but particularly from the Relationship centre of X (another mind). We feel the best path is to eliminate the reproductive function, this is due to the guilt and shame X experiences in the relationship centre. There is the complication of pleasure and joy as well, but we weigh this up."

"So are you referring to some kind of a necrotic tendency based on perceptions of guilt and shame being acted upon"?

"Yes, the guilt is of the kind related to being seen having pleasure related to sex, it has the energy of hiding and yet continuing in the face of the fear of exposure."

"How do the feelings of pleasure play into this? Also there is the aspect of reproductive urge to consider as well?"

"We hear all of that too, but these messages are not as strong"

"Can you help to resolve things so that communication is more clear and together we can release the pattern of being which includes the psychology, and overgrowth conditions? and if so we request that you help us to resolve this so that the suffering of X can be relieved"

"We can show a way. To progress we, the Candida, need good access to all of the psychology of X, then we need to assist the relationship mind to be clear about guilty or shameful feelings, bring these out of the subconscious and out into the conscious, and to release these progressively. We need to be clear between us that that there is also the pleasure and reproductive urge, and that this also has weight. To do this the Relationship centre needs the support of the other minds."

They continue – "I show you now the two aspects of the relationship centre (masculine and feminine) standing in the centre of the circle and all 8 other relationship mind aspects standing around holding hands. We, the Candida, are standing with these minds too and acting like a web of information flow around the entire system, and the information flowing is love and understanding for the suffering of the relationship centre aspects, and for the suffering of x's body. The experience is like a prayer, so we refer to what you and X refer to as the higher principles relating to X as well. Our Hive will communicate this to other organisms too."

I as practitioner then facilitated the implementation of this collaborative approach.

As an afterword, the client reported some weeks later that the fungal aspect had resolved completely, however there remained some skin issues – I asked the Candida what was happening. The reply was that there was a localised population of Staphylococcus creating the residual overgrowth conditions. The Candida and I talked to this population, which it turned out was a residue of sexual contact from decades ago, and so was not the same strain as the rest of the Staphylococcus in the body. This residual strain after more than 20 years still felt like an outsider and was very fearful and so was "dug in" The Candida assisted me to show it the diversity of the microbiome, and that it was a welcome addition to it. There was a release of the belief systems and the fear.

Case Study 2 - Female middle age - distressed sacral area with severe pain and some immobilisation

I introduced the situation – "We have been doing consciousness work with your host body and your Hive-mind and also other organisms, the focus of that work was largely to move the balance points so that the body of your host can be healthier in general. That work most recently was in most part around appetite and the sense of satiation or fullness. As soon as we did this work the hosts sacral area became severely distressed, including an apparent misalignment of the left side sacroiliac joint. This experience was noted when the hosts body was sitting normally in a chair. It seems more than coincidental. Do you have anything to say to us so we may better understand what happened? Do you have suggestions to resolve this and how we should proceed?"

You will recall that we together (host, Hive-mind, and Neil) had identified that the nervous signalling from the smooth musculature of the stomach, and also all of the small and large intestines was being limited. We also note that we the Candida of the body were directly involved with this. We were acting on instructions around making sure that the body was well stocked up with fat in case there was a future limitation on access to food.

We felt the need to store away ever larger quantities of energy in the form of body fat.

We acted directly on this by limiting the nervous signalling efficiency so that the host was always hungry no matter how full the digestive system was.

The therapy process clearly showed us two things, one was that there is no shortage of stored energy, there is no risk to the host body nor to the Hive organisms, there is plenty of stored energy. Also, that the host has no need be fearful in this area.

The Candida organisms in the sacral area also acted upon this general call to remove interference with pain or pressure receptors and released their influence over the signalling of the pain receptor nerves. They too were previously responding to nourishment of another kind and the fear of a lack of it. Here it related to the being nourished emotionally by the hosts father starting at about the age of 11. Since that time we have been modifying the effectiveness of the pain receptors, We have done this at the hosts request."

The therapy after this included the emotional release from the pelvic region of the fears associated with this long-standing experience of the client (Host)

Case 3 – Male Middle Aged - shoulder issue, with pain associated with movement and lack of range of movement. Non repair of shoulder injuries after an event of a fall some six months earlier.

"The muscles of the shoulder of your host were injured due to a fall, I sense that the failure to repair more quickly is due to a subtle impediment, do you the Candida Hive-mind have any information to share that may help us understand this situation, and can we work together to reach an early repair to the shoulder?"

"The host has spent years with this right masculine shoulder trying to effect feminine outcomes. We have closed off the effect of the web of our Hive from the region to try to assist the host to resolve this."

"So you have merely stopped being involved?"

"We are providing information to the host through the withdrawal of our attempts to cover things over, this host has many resources at his disposal to work through these matters; we see clearly the confusion in this case. He is trying to manage what he perceives as continuous hostility from the environment in a feminine way with a structure which has strong masculine predilections. That shoulder would inevitably attract an injury or a disease representing this confusion. Our only direct involvement is in the creation of scar tissue, we have supported this to create less movement."

Therapy was to assist the Client (host) throughout their being to understand the processes involved in this misapplication of the consciousness of the shoulders, and to suggest the appropriate repairs to the affected tissues. These new arrangements included the relationships of the two shoulders, the spinal brain and the thoracic brain and the masculine and feminine mind aspects of these two physical brains.

Case study 4 – Adult Male - Putting on Weight – Belief System that "I am my own worst enemy"

I have done much research into the consciousness of healthy weight. Including the development of my TRIM program which is a suggestion-based program you can use at home. (Currently being redeveloped to utilise the coherence device)

Recently I had a client for whom there were still road blocks to success. I had this person on my Coherence device, and thought to ask the Candida, which has many scientifically evidenced involvements around appetite and fat physiology and metabolism in particular, what it had to offer on why the person was still holding weight despite other work done and much care taken with diet and exercise.

The answer was complex with metabolic processes at the fore. Interestingly however the Candida was involved in supporting these misguided metabolic actions.

I asked why it was participating. The answer was it was responding to a dominant belief system. The belief system was that "I am my own worst enemy" This belief system is general within this person, so covering everything from success in the world of work, and also in relationships, and also in all of the matters that affect his health. So the concept being acted on here is that he is hurting himself repeatedly, and that he is guilty of purposeful and wilful damage etc etc.

As mentioned earlier, the Candida Hive-mind does not distinguish clearly between the cells of the body, and the cells of all of the microbes, including the Candida. To them it is all "Us" so this strong belief system of the human leads the Hive-mind to belief that it is the organisms worst enemy. A belief that is strongly reinforced by the continuous deluge of consciousness about the "Bad Disease Organisms"

All of the resultant efforts by the Candida to manipulate the behaviour of the general physiology flow on from this, and the direct interruption of processes around holding or releasing fat occur. The Candida was literally acting out the part in the play where it was the villain. It was assisting metabolism which ensured the stopping of the release of fats so that that needed energy would be available for cell use, and on top of this was assisting in the creation of false appetites, especially appetites for energy dense foods.

The therapy was to reassure the Candida that it is not the root of all evil. Particularly that it could stop acting as though it were. The new approach could be to encourage the balanced functioning of fat storage and release of fats into the sugar metabolism as the new priority. There is no need for it to micromanage the perception that the client is wilfully overeating, far better for the client to realise by normal feedback that they are in fact full or indeed hungry as the case may be. And lastly for there to be no feelings of guilt around this, and that without this complexity the client can make better conscious mind level choices.

Case Study 5 – Female Middle Aged – Ankle Injury not healing.

Client with persistent scar tissue in the ligaments and tendons/muscles around a joint, despite the careful application of physically based therapeutic treatment, along with care with nutrition, added to other energetic therapy support for the repair of the joint. The scar tissue is non-aligned connective tissue, which forms subsequent to an accident to act like a splint to support the repairing tissues. Under normal conditions it naturally would dissolve away once the joint tissues were repaired after an injury. This kind of disabling presentation isn't uncommon. We commonly see people who say, had an injury in their twenties, and now in their forties the injury seemingly hasn't "gone away". So we ask what is there from a consciousness perspective that is leading to the decision not to dissolve away this tissue.

So we meet again with our microflora, They persistently hear the information that we are an injured person in this particular joint. (All joints have a consciousness persistently associated- in this case it is an ankle which has many consciousness but one of them is around walking straight, and or, perhaps in another direction.)

So the microbes are hearing. "I cant keep focussed, I can't find my way in life – I am easily distracted, along with the belief, I am unsupported in my endeavours" They respond by retaining these beliefs in this joint. They communicate with the scar tissue cells in the ankle and support them in the decision at the time of cell division to persist in this disorganised tissue rather than allowing the cell death and encouragement of the coordinated tissues to form.

We decided to form a Tetra to work with this. In this tetra the virus has the information needed and the ability to deliver this information into the cell nucleus, the bacteria have the ability to pre-digest the cell that no longer supports the intention of the body and it's minds, and the fungi the skills to further digest it and also, of far more vital importance, the skills and opportunity to also manage the coordination of the whole process of reorganisation at the cellular level, including the coordination, along with the moving centre (mind level – so macro understanding of how the joint should perform), of the host to ensure the applicable new laying down of coordinated well-adjusted tissues. This last comes as the Moving Centre decides on action around those beliefs we mentioned earlier.

In therapy what is needed is for the host/client and or therapist to witness or observe all of this, and to affirm to all of the parties that the tissues no longer need to be based in their structure and organisation on these old belief systems. The Coherence device helps in this observation and also with the affirmations, but it is far from essential. The capacity to clearly and with focus observe is really all that is needed.

In our case here as a result of this observation the client's ankle is improving daily. Seems like a miracle, until you realise its just a cooperative project of a virus, a bacteria, a fungi and the human cells guided by a relatively coherent mind of the host.

This opportunity exists for us all.

Case Study 6 – Male, middle-aged and wildly fluctuating between over-weight, and something that could be described as a more natural-weight.

Here the specific tissues are the external adipose tissues, in this case nearly all of it situated around the abdomen and thorax. So we are not talking here of the fat situated around organs, rather we are talking about the fat outside of most of the body's musculature

A little bit of background here, this kind of weight in this client is made up of three major components, firstly there are the fat cells themselves. These are like fuel tanks, where the metabolic business of the cell occurs in a corner of the cell and the balance of the cell is a cavity which can fill up or empty out of fats. Then there are the extracellular fluids. This is mainly a water like fluid with a mixture of salts, and also metabolites. There are a reasonable quantity of cells, including immune cells, floating around in this too. It can be considered as an aspect of the lymph, but whereas most lymph is busy moving from one place to another, this fluid is more static, it is like a reservoir of water. The last aspect of this so-called surplus weight is the supporting structure. This is a pretty solid tissue and is often a very difficult tissue type for a dieter to eliminate from their body.

This client has a wide fluctuation in the fluid held around the tissue cells and the fat stored in each fat cell can fluctuate pretty widely and quickly too. The structural material is more static.

The consciousness of the host in general can fluctuate around the question of the purpose for their own existence and has energetic forays into sadness and a feeling of depletion and a sense of the "pointlessness of it all". It is this consciousness that is acting right within these tissues.

So the minds involved here include the emotional, and the instinctive, and the moving centres as follows. The Emotional centre is involved in the sadness, and the resultant separation that attaches to loneliness too. The instinctive centre is involved in yo-yo actions of the storage system and a type of stagnation and slowness around adaptation. The Moving Centre is involved in the actions of either energetically encouraging movement of all stored contents, or alternately something that looks a bit like lethargic tendencies where there is a huge lag in acting on the intentions of the Instinctive Centre.

In this client's case higher up the hierarchy in the human, there is a fluctuation around hope and hopelessness. Will he naturally succeed in life or does he give up?

We would, in therapy, normally tend to work at this top level with the psychology. But consider now how many steps of psychology we are away from the intersection with the interactions with the Candida. And to add to it consider how many minds are involved too. Just to be clear the Candida organisms can be involved in intercepting all of the biology here, so what the Candida Hive-mind is intending is vital to the outcome.

So to get the intentions of the macro human to be coherent with the inherited intentions of the Candida Hive-mind we have to tidy all of this up.

The treatment is to observe all of this, get it out in the open, as a very important and "weighty piece of evidence" for the Hive-mind to be able to utilise as part of their assessment of the "weight of evidence".

Meanwhile the Candida living in and around these specific tissues can monitor the actions of these minds in the tissues and report it to the rest of the Hive's cells. They can see the shift of these minds based on the new intentions coming from a desire to shift consciousness. Based on this weight of evidence, the Candida situated in the neurological tissues in each physical brain can support shifts in the neurochemistry to support the mind activity towards these new intentions. Similarly the Candida situated in the major tissues of the hormonal system can also encourage new balances of hormonal signalling as well, all directed at shifting the mood component support of the minds.

The outcome here is far more coherent action, the minds are concerted in their action, there is far less confusion, the hormonal chemistry and neurochemistry supports a more active and proactive model of behaviour, so are supporting a more positive outlook, this in turn supports all of the processes right down to activation and re-balancing of the fluid quantities, leading finally to a stabilised more-healthy body weight.

Case Study 7 – Male Senior. Viral infection.

Replication Process of any viral infection Driven by the Host Cells vs. by the Virus

In this case, a patient was experiencing an unseasonal head cold with some additional flu like symptoms. The case occurred over the Southern Hemisphere summer 2019/2020 as the corona virus fears were emerging.

So I asked the virus was it the corona virus. There was nothing in reply. I showed the virus the fear and panic in the world community about this new C-19 variant of the long known more general corona virus. The virus said it was the old sort. Not the variant.

I told the patient they should see a doctor in case this self-diagnostic information from the virus needed a second opinion ☺.

We proceeded to look at the information the virus had for the host. Again this information was sketchy. I felt the information was far from being freely shared. So I asked for support from the wider microbial community. The Candida came forward and showed me the fear response in the virus. The virus wasn't sure it could share safely, because it felt everything was trying to eliminate it along with the c-19 virus which is it's cousin. This fear was causing all of these viruses to become extremely prolific, to say nothing of developing an almost paranoiac behaviour set.

With reassurance, through us showing the virus that it was a part of a wide community of viruses in the body, and generally that we did not seek to eliminate it. Further trust was created by highlighting the benefits to the host which would be achieved by the already diverse viral stock within the host's body. Eventually there came a relaxation in the virus.

The Candida continued as a bridge agent. Showing the original emotional climate that led to the virus activating a growth process. It was based on a strong feeling of sadness (subclinical depression). This was made more urgent by the host becoming frustrated, a kind of anger response the next day.

The therapy was to show all of this clearly amongst physiological suggestions to the body of the host. We identified that the virus had a role to play but that didn't mean it had to reproduce to such numbers that the host would have to respond through illness. We asked the Candida to assist in the translation of all this information.

Another important component in the therapy was that the hosts immune system collaborated with this microbe led approach. Here, under the direction of the microbes, the immune processes were given clear information as to the nature of the virus. The immune system was able to see the virus very quickly and create the antigen. The microbes coordinated the delivery of these antigens to the appropriate sites. They shared the information with the host cells where replication of the virus was occurring.

Of more importance the microbes delivered the information to the host cells so that they understood the collaborative goal of not reproducing such vast numbers of the virus particles.

This led to a very streamlined approach to lessening the scale and rate of the replication of the virus.

To be clear. The strategy for lessening the symptoms of the overgrowth of the virus was driven by the microbes. Once commenced the actual replication processes are far more driven by the host cells than they are by the virus itself. Therefore, the action needed to come mainly from the host side of the equation.

The resultant lessening in symptoms was immediate.

(Note I have a forthcoming book on working with viruses – The working title is "Beautiful Information")

Case Study 8 – Male – issues with creating abundance

Emphasizing the Role of the Relationship Mind.

The client and his partner have been looking to establish themselves in a more abundant setting, but they find themselves looking at more of a scarcity-based model. This includes financial issues but the energy crosses into other areas of their lives too such as finding that many opportunities are always just a little out of their reach.

The client is situated in Europe, and I am in Australia, so the treatment was of the distance intention type. I was hooked up to the coherence device in Perth, Australia and the client was on skype and in a meditative state sitting on a balcony overlooking the Sea.

The therapy commenced with focus on the Super Conscious level of the Yang aspect of the Relationship centre (Mind). The opportunity was to widely open up the relationship centre to receive and to give communication. The energy here was that he could reach out in an almost unlimited fashion to the environment. What he is doing as this treatment is being installed is broadcasting a message that says "I am here and I wish to collaborate". At the same time he is dramatically increasing his perception, so is also broadcasting a message that says "I am listening".

The Relationship centre does also have a role in reproduction of course.

However the huge majority of the Relationship Mind's function is to manage the 7 c's:

- ✓ Contact
- ✓ Connection
- ✓ Communication
- ✓ Commonality
- ✓ Cooperation
- ✓ Collaboration
- ✓ Coherence

The relationship mind is absolutely pivotal in the management of this progression. In this first part of the treatment we are encouraging the master controller of the interactions with the environment to use its highest mind level of functioning to reach out to the environment. The super conscious of the relationship centre/mind is closely aligned to the subtle functioning of the Brow and Crown Chakras too, so these high level environment seeking Chakras are also involved in this aspect of the therapy.

The Candida then showed us how to proceed. They showed the benefits of the flat non-hierarchical structure that defines the Candida Hive-mind. They showed resources in their true state of unlimited availability. They gave us the image of a gentle tidal wave of resources flowing towards us, an endless flow of energy. This flow was coming into the client via the superconscious of the Yang aspect of the Relationship centre. It is interesting that it is the Yang aspect. There was no clarity in the treatment as to why this was. However we can assume for this client it is needed to focus Yang in order to move towards more balance.

The next thing the Candida showed us was how to go about the distribution of this abundant energy. The flow was to firstly process this through the Instinctive Centre predominantly in the Subconscious, both Yin and Yang.

Here there was a couple of barriers to the flow. They were epigenetic, relating to many ancestors, but predominantly ones who were having active experiences around the end of the Second World War.

The belief systems that centred here were ones of having to watch our backs in case someone else comes and takes away our money. So it is a conservative mindset that limits being open in any way.

I discussed this with the client and he reassured me that this was exactly how he felt. That if he did things for another person that as a result his energy was depleted. The Candida Hive-mind gave me the metaphorical thumbs up and we continued.

Having established a program to release the epigenetic limitations focussed in the subconscious of the instinctive mind/centre we moved onto the continuation of the flow of this abundance.

The next area was the Conscious Mind Yang aspect of the Moving Centre. The Moving Centre has many unconscious roles in the body including coordination of many aspects of physiological function. In the conscious mind where we are looking it is in part about planning and taking practical action.

The Candida showed examples of the unusual and unexpected desire to make a phone call or to reach out to someone through social media. The energy here is a very practical, and no nonsense, Yang approach. The treatment showed a way past any fears of taking action and the possibility for rejection.

The next thing the Candida showed was the movement of this abundance wave into the Emotional Mind/Centre. In this case to the Yin aspect of the Sub-of-the-Subconscious aspect of the Emotional Centre.

This is the deepest area of our minds, completely hidden from our conscious minds view. In here we were shown barriers too. These barriers were around allowing Love and Compassion for people who are struggling to find resources.

There was a linkage to the ancestors we mentioned earlier, but critically it was to show how the client can change things to then be able to have compassion for the suffering of those around him right now. The particular suffering is the need to compete, and to jealously hold onto resources, rather than the alternate nature to share and collaborate.

Once this was established as a new mode of operation, the Candida showed how this could be applied to the Self as well. So deep Sub-of-the-Sub-Conscious Emotional Centre love of self and Compassion for anything within self that limits openness.

After this we were shown the open flow of the endless wave of abundance, through every aspect of the client, and on and out into the environment to enrich everything it comes into contact with.

There were many other aspects of the therapy, however my purpose in sharing here was to highlight the extent to which the Candida, and the Candida Hive-mind were willing and capable to assist their Host. Of course, my Candida were participating too.

This case study shows an exceptionally high level of Collaboration between the intention of the Host, and the Host Mind aspects, and the Hive-mind. In this case there is no Candida involvement in disease presentation at all, and yet the Candida openly and willingly participated in this high-level therapy.

Case Study 9 - Domesticated Cat – Profound issues with Gut Health and Complex interactions with Humans.

This Case study follows on from a variety of earlier sessions I have provided for this Cat and also for the human that lives with him.

The request for the therapy seemingly came from this cat.

I was on the coherence device in my clinic in Australia, and on a call to the human associated with the cat as well. They live in another country in an inner city apartment environment.

The Cat (x) had overheard an earlier conversation and treatment I had done for x's human. In that treatment there were references to how cats can elect to form communities with humans under those situations where they are allowed to do so by the human. In these cases, the places (usually a home) become as much a cat place as they are human place. X was wanting to explore what this all meant in the context of his own life.

As a side note - The process of animal and for that matter microbial communication involved in this case study and the rest of this book occurs when the human allows it. It involves a purposeful five minds-based disorientation.

The people who are naturals in this arena are usually in the Autism Spectrum. Not all spectrum people can do this, but a surprising number with practice can. I refer you to my book "Unleashing your Autism Superpowers" for more detail on the superpower of animal communication.

On the other side of the communication is the animal themselves and they are able to borrow aspects of the processing of the human so that they can hold up their end of the conversation. The Microbial Hives do this as well.

In this session I was purposefully opening up as many of the aspects of my processing and memories as I could. X's human who was on a call with me during this session was also intentionally doing this as well.

X was a part of a very large litter, where the mother cat had struggled to feed all of the kittens. The cat could be thought of as the runt of the litter.

X's human who in their terms in effect "rescued" X from his previous human (this human had earlier "rescued" X from the original human associated with the litter, shared their strongly held opinion with us that X today is responding to earlier fear around his experience and feels fear about the possibility of returning to the scarcity in his upbringing.

X's human also detailed what in their view was extreme trauma for X.

The perceived trauma related to an unusual situation where hungry kittens will sometime try to suckle on the other kittens and this can include the penises of the male kittens. X had had this experience, and in the process had been bitten which led to the need for repeated surgery on his penis. This all was equated as trauma for X.

The extent and power of the held view of this perceived trauma which was described as the "Abuse" that X was subjected too were now held as powerful beliefs in the five minds of the human.

This is an important component in this therapy.

This interaction was overheard by X. He was puzzled so we took some time to explore this.

X's memory seemed to vary. He didn't feel traumatised by the shortfall of food, nor the inappropriate, in the human context, attention of the other kittens. He did however feel quite traumatised by the experience with the vet and the surgery.

X's human discussed some maladapted behaviours in the eyes of the earlier human he was associated with. These maladaptive behaviours led this human to be very angry with X. This anger was sited as further trauma for X.

X was certainly aware of the anger, but hadn't joined the dots with the perceived maladaptive behaviour.

As another side note, I do a lot of animal communication as a part of my therapy work. Some topics are completely no-go areas for some animals. These in my observation relate to what the animal feels is completely natural behaviour.

So as an example if a dog is a digging type of dog then talking about this with the dog as being maladaptive behaviour has almost no impact on their behaviour. They just don't have the cognition of what the problem is. You can retrain the dog at this point, however it still makes no sense to the dog.

In this case from the time of retraining on for the dog this is now a nice and pleasant experience (digging) that they are no longer allowed to pursue.

I suspect we are in the same kind of territory with this early kitten experience and the behaviour of his siblings towards X. To the human it looks like the other kittens abused X and for that matter it was sexual abuse. To X the behaviour of the other kittens was relatively normal, and not of itself traumatising.

X suffers from acute diarrhoea and has done so since well before X came to live with his current human. The extent of this does vary over time but it remains persistent. I was interested to find out the patterns for this, and as X had called for the session due to his concern at the distress that his human experienced around this diarrhoea I felt we were near the real point of the session.

X's Human spoke about how they had gotten together. X was not adapted to where he was living in a rescue shelter setting. They made a very deep connection upon first meeting and X went home with his human that first day.

X's human expressed their observation that there was resonance between the trauma of X and their own trauma. And that this trauma was persistent throughout the period of each of their lives leading up to the adoption.

As the therapy continued it was increasingly clear that the context of X's perception and memory was quite different to the context of either myself as therapist, and most importantly also the context of X's human.

The Candida Hive of X now wished to be heard and a conversation was opened up with it and X and X's human.

The Hive agreed with my queries around the timing and origins of the microbial balance changes in X's colon. It cited a specific change in the choices being acted upon at the time of the surgeries. These choices were the encouragement of very definite strategies within X's body generally and in the colon in particular.

The Hive continued to outline the ways in which the five minds states of the previous humans associated with X and critically also the five minds state of the vet as well, had been used as data supporting the decision.

X showed then how as the runt of the litter he was attracting attention by being demanding. The demanding behaviour was annoying to the humans and led to significant anger. This was confusing because the humans were also expressing love and good will towards X as well.

In all of this experience there is the germination of a victim mentality. Largely the humans have originated this, and then X perpetuates that part of it that is consistent with his own experience.

His experience is one of quite severe physical suffering, as well as the psychological experience.

The Hive is responding to this mixed information. They are balancing all of this data and arising to the top of the pile of data is the potent nature of the disgust of the humans around the injury to X's penis. This disgust was a significant or as I describe it "weighted" factor.

Today many years later the Hive has retained it's own memories of this data event. *The hive showed how they utilised the tissues of the colon* (nearest tissue to the largest population density of the hives cells within the body of X) *to store their own memories of the experience.* These memories are added to X's memories as well.

The topic of desexing of domestic animals was raised by the Hive, they were seeking more detail from me, so I showed the concepts of population pressure, and available resources, and the then often followed human decisions based on these matters including desexing these animals. The Hive could not grasp this at all from it's own perspective of how the microbial community operates. For the hive the life or death of the individual cell was completely natural to it.

The hive had made the connection between desexing a cat, and the surgeries, and the horror of the humans around the injuries to X's penis in the first place. All of this complexity is being added as weighty data.

I summarised my understanding of the confusion for both X and the Hive. A confused setting where there is five minds' data coming to the Hive from a range of humans and also from X himself.

I asked the hive what source and which particular data was the most weighted.

They replied the evidence being supplied by X was highest but followed and reinforced by that from the Humans.

We are therefore looking at a situation where the psychology of the humans affects the psychology of the cat, and then this in turn is most important in the impact on what we might think of as the psychology of the Hive.

The Hive acknowledge this nested relationship. I showed the Hive the metaphor of Russian dolls where a doll is nested inside another doll etc. A metaphor which was helpful to the Hive.

We then began to examine the impact of all of these psychological matters onto the overall equation.

X's human spoke about their anger at abusive men who had impacted on their own life. They reflected that the anger along with other emotional responses had been very strong at different times during the association of them with X.

We therefore enquired of X and the Hive into their experience when encountering this type of anger. They both agreed that this was observed in real time and factored into the equation by both the minds of X and also the Hive.

X's human discussed the confusion between X as a male cat and roles of men who had impacted on their life. X agreed that he felt this and cried for their suffering.

The Hive made the observation that their action was also tied to this. However the processes were very confusing for the Hive. Even so they could identify that the attempt to wipe out the villi of the colon which is the structural outcome of the choices made in influencing microflora balance in the colon was related to this.

There is in this choice a variation of the intention of castrating men.

At this point in the therapy It became clear that an overall microbiome Hive mind was participating as well. It was clear that X and the nested Hives and X's Human were all now participating in resolving long standing suffering and trauma.

Further the desire to do this had been set at the time that X met his human. The therapy in a sense was operating across or outside of the gap of linear time.

The implementation was the release of the emasculatory tendencies that had burdened the microbiome generally. This was a release of the need that led to choices for microbial population densities which led on to the degradation and finally the acute inflammatory response, and subsequent leaking into the bloodstream of the villi of the colon walls.

The therapy covered many details encouraging a gradient of available access for the microbes going from the colon contents side of the villi to the blood side of it.

As a part of this release there is the opportunity for the Yin and Yang aspects of all participants to be met, honoured, and then allowed to harmonise. The duality needs to be fully experienced before the jump to unity can occur.

The final message arising in this therapy relates to the role of the humans involved in this and other cases involving humans and other beings on the planet. The humans have an opportunity for choice at a far greater scale than other beings, and the responsibility of the sovereign human is to make choices that further the 7 c's that lead finally to coherence between all beings.

We humans have the gift of choice. We can choose coherence between ourselves and all other beings here on earth.

All we need do is accept this role of being the

maker of choices.

Contents

www.ingramcontent.com/pod-product-compliance
Lightning Source LLC
Chambersburg PA
CBHW020913180526
45163CB00007B/2711